Miracles from the Other Side

How My Near-Death Experience Saved My Life

Heather Vandermeyden

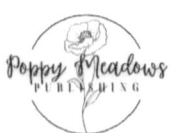

Poppy Meadows
PUBLISHING

Contents

Praise for Miracles from the Other Side

As a person who has walked the path of the afterlife and returned, I can tell you that Heather Vandermeyden's *Miracles from the Other Side* is not just a book—it's a journey into the unseen realms of life, death, and the soul's eternal purpose. Through Heather's beautifully written words, we are given an intimate and profoundly moving account of her near-death experience, one filled with wisdom, comfort, and extraordinary clarity.

I have witnessed firsthand the immense power of a transformative spiritual experience, and in Heather's story, I felt a kindred connection to what I, too, encountered on the other side. The way Heather describes her out-of-body experience—the peace, the overwhelming love, the lack of fear, and the deep understanding that transcends our earthly concerns—will resonate deeply with anyone who has questioned what truly happens when we cross over.

Heather's words are a testament to the beauty of the afterlife and the boundless love that exists beyond this physical world. *Miracles from the Other Side* is not only a book about death; it is a guide to living more fully, more consciously, and more connected to the divine. Her words are imbued with the kind of truth that only comes from having touched the eternal.

This book is a gift to all seeking answers to life's biggest questions. Heather shares her personal journey with such grace and vulnerability that it becomes impossible to not be moved. I am deeply honored to endorse *Miracles from the Other Side*, knowing that it will touch many hearts and bring healing and peace to those who read it. Heather has opened a window to the other side, and through her story, we see that love and light are the greatest miracles of all.

May Heather's words guide you to a deeper understanding of the miracles that await us all on the other side of this life.

— Jeffery Olsen
Speaker and Author of *Knowing*

Miracles from the Other Side is a book that takes a fresh look at near-death experiences (NDEs) from the unique perspective of the author, Heather Vandermeyden. It begins with the intense details of the day in January 2000 when Heather died in the hospital. As her soul left her body, although aware of the frantic medical efforts by doctors and nurses to save her life, she felt peace and exhilaration at the prospect of dying. Why? She had already undergone several surgeries, experienced intense pain, and was nearing the end of her capacity to endure.

From this intense beginning, the book moves back to an earlier time in Heather's life, from which it then takes the reader through the events and traumas that led up to her surgery. The reader is told how Heather learned she would adopt two children, how she instantly knew who they were, and how she came to know and love them.

During one of her NDEs, Heather heard lovely, heavenly music and experienced what she describes as healing waters on the other side—elements not often found in NDEs. With elegance, charm, and some humor, Heather describes her many trials, interwoven with her awareness of angels ministering to hospital patients and seeing orbs that were somehow family members who had long since passed on.

Heather describes popping in and out of her physical body—essentially, a series of NDEs. She also experienced another less common element in NDEs: being told that certain memories she had of the other side would be forgotten to prevent certain purposes of her life from being thwarted.

Miracles from the Other Side is a delightful, thoughtful, well-written book, which will no doubt be popular and read by many.

—Martin Tanner, BA, JD, Vice President and Member of the Board of
Directors IANDS, Cofounder
Utah IANDS, Radio Talk Show Host and Podcaster

Miracles from the Other Side is a story of severe health challenges laced with beautifully descriptive and frequent visits to the other side. The ride is compelling as Heather skillfully describes the beauty and freedoms of heaven and then drops us back into an earth-body filled with unfathomable pain and weakness. I fell in love with Heather's fiery spunk as she filled her pockets with rocks to create positive hospital weigh-ins. *Miracles* is full of unique, dry humor and laugh-out-loud observations, and serves as a testimony of the continuation of life after life and the possibility that any one of us can be still and hear the promptings from the Other Side as we develop a personal relationship with our Spirit Guides.

—Claudia Watts Edge, Author of Award-Winning
Gifts from the Edge, Lessons from the Edge, and *We Touched Heaven*

Inspiring, heartwarming, awestruck, endurance. Words that come to mind after reading this book. As you read about the severity of Heather's illness, where she teetered between two worlds, one that brought her peace and comfort, one that caused her intense pain, be prepared for the ups and downs of your emotions. In Heather's story, you will be laughing one minute and gasping the next as she shares the vivid details of how her physical body became so sick she wanted to give up. The space she experienced when she was out of consciousness tempted her with a more beautiful life. Torn between these experiences and messages she received about her earthly existence, she continued to fight unimaginable circumstances so that she could receive the blessings that awaited her physical state. This story is a testament to how our bodies can be taken through extreme illnesses, barely functioning, yet with proper care, patience, hard work, and time, bounce back so that a young woman could become the mother and daughter she was intended to be. Not only did Heather survive her ordeal, but she also finds reason to laugh in every day she is given.

—Wendy L Hooton, #1 International Best-Selling Author,
Speaker, Down Syndrome Advocate

Heather's story is more than a near-death experience—it's a sacred transmission of Light, Hope, and Remembrance. Her words carry the kind of truth that stirs the soul and opens the heart to what is eternal. I've known Heather for years, and the wisdom she offers through this book is the same quiet, radiant presence she brings to everyone she touches. This is not just a book; it's a gift, a healing, and a homecoming.

—Vincent "Vinney" Todd Tolman, Near-Death Experience Survivor, Author of *The Light After Death*, and Inspirational Speaker

Library of Congress Control Number: 2025908041

Cover Design by Francine Eden Platt of Eden Graphics, Inc

Interior Layout by Robert Harrison of Seneca Author Services

Publisher–Poppy Meadows Publishing

Salt Lake City, Utah

ISBN 979-8-89454-062-7 (Paperback)

ISBN 979-8-89454-072-6 (Hardcover)

www.heathervandermeyden.com

What Happens When We Die?

As our soul gently separates from our body, we enter a realm more beautiful than words in any language can describe. This place radiates with immense love, profound peace, and joy so complete it transcends earthly understanding. We are instantly freed from pain, illness, and every burden we carried in life. We are made whole again.

In this sacred space, we are welcomed by loved ones who passed before us, their happiness at our reunion wrapping us in warmth and familiarity. We gain deep insights into life, the universe, and our divine purpose. We discover we are fully known—every thought, every moment—and unconditionally loved.

This experience surpasses even the most cherished moments of our lives. Earth, with all its beauties and hardships, has served as our class-room. Now, having completed our lessons, we return to the home we left behind—the place where our soul has always belonged.

Dedication

This book would not exist without my mother—my anchor, my light, and my quiet strength. She carried me through the darkest storms. No mother should ever have to stand at the edge of the unknown, watching her child slip between life and death, powerless to intervene. And yet she did—with grace; fierce, unwavering love; and a heart vast enough to hold both hope and heartbreak.

Mom, you carried my pain as if it were your own, wrapping me in grace when I had none to offer, always placing my needs above your own and asking nothing in return. Your love is the reason I am still here. It is the kind that heals, the kind that endures, the kind that saves.

You are the quiet miracle behind every word in these pages, the steady hand behind my healing, the sacred presence that called me back when I was nearly gone. Without you, I would not be here to tell this story. You are my hero, my best friend, and the soul to whom these pages are lovingly devoted.

This is for you, Mom—with all my love.

Foreword

I met twenty-year-old Heather Vandermeyden in December 1999 when she arrived in my emergency department. Her heart raced to support her sagging blood pressure. Her blood tests were concerning. I initiated her resuscitation and admitted her to the hospital.

I knew she was critically ill, but I didn't know then about *the voice*.

Twenty-five years later, Heather found me and told me the rest of her story. Weeks before we met in the ER, she'd heard a masculine voice. "You'll be dying soon," it had whispered in a strangely comforting tone, "and there's nothing to be afraid of."

Heather soon found herself in an intensive care unit on a ventilator and unable to speak because of the tube in her throat. The first time she left her body, she watched from an elevated position as medical professionals worked to resuscitate her. She was so sick for so long that she left her body repeatedly and sometimes, outside her physical form, left the hospital to check on family.

While she hovered between realms, Heather saw angels comforting patients. And when patients died, those unseen angels gathered and consoled the grieving families.

When Heather stood at the entrance of heaven, she saw a path lined with beings of light. She knew it led to her deceased grandmother, and she knew she wasn't permitted to go. "It's not your time," she was told. Still, she asked to see her grandmother but immediately found herself back in her body instead.

On multiple occasions, two blond-haired, hazel-eyed children, a boy and a girl, appeared at Heather's bedside, sometimes accompanied by an elderly man. Heather spoke about the children with her mother, but her mother could never see them. Years later, Heather's anticipations found fulfillment when she adopted the children who visited her in the hospital.

Heather's peaceful demeanor belied the severity of her illness during our first encounter, but when we met again twenty-five years later, the same peaceful demeanor witnessed to the verity of what she shared. Science can't explain such experiences, but I know they are real because I've had them myself. I've seen souls leave their bodies in the emergency department, and they've communicated with me after their physical death.

I'm grateful Heather came into my life. And I'm grateful she is sharing her story.

—Jeff O'Driscoll, MD, Spiritual Mentor, Author, Speaker, and Artist

A Note from the Author

Dear Reader,

January of 2025 marked twenty-five years since my soul left my body during a medical crisis and I experienced life on the Other Side. I have never felt it was the right time to share my story until now. While it was an incredibly personal experience, I hope my words can reach and comfort those who fear death or believe that when we die, we simply cease to exist.

My near-death experience, or NDE, transformed and humbled me in a way that is hard to put into words, but I will do my best.

I was fortunate to have copies of my medical records, bills, journals, and family members' recollections to rely on for details, like diagnosis names and surgery dates, while writing this book. They brought clarity to a chapter of my life that felt fragmented and overwhelming. But it was still freshly painful, still emotionally hard to look back on those awful days and remember how critically ill I was during my hospitalization. I should not be alive, but I am. While I wish I could take back or forget the physical pain I endured, I have no regrets. I know this was part of my path. This ordeal changed the course of my life and gifted me with a knowledge that there is truly another existence after we leave this Earth.

Each of us is known and loved by Our Creator. The afterlife is more wonderful and magical than we can imagine in even our wildest dreams. I look forward to the day when I can return home once again and reunite with loved ones who patiently await my return.

Chapter 1

The Doorway Between Worlds

I died on Wednesday, January 12, 2000.

From a quiet corner of the room, I watched my nurses fight desperately to pull me back, voices pleading, as my soul drifted peacefully away from the chaos. In that breathtaking moment, I felt more alive than ever. I experienced a beautiful, exquisite stillness beyond pain and fear—a moment where time seemed to dissolve and the true essence of life revealed itself. It was as if I had been touched by something eternal, bathed in a light beyond this world, cradled by a profound peace that whispered love, purpose, and divine grace.

To everyone else, it was a crisis; to me, it was a sacred space—a quiet homecoming my spirit longed for. It felt as though I was being gently welcomed back to a place I always knew but somehow forgot, where there was no fear or pain—only peace, light, and a love that encircled me like a familiar embrace. Everyone in the room did whatever they could to keep me alive, valiantly struggling with medical equipment and my useless body, their anxiety and worry crowding out all other thoughts. But I was already gone, watching from the Other Side, suspended in stillness, untouched by the panic, wrapped in a peace so profound it felt like I had slipped beyond the reach of suffering itself. As machines beeped in the background, I wished everyone would stop the frantic efforts, stop fighting for a body I no longer belonged to, and just let me go home. Home to my real home —heaven. I felt no connection to that limp body lying there, no connection to their worry about it. If anything, I felt a detached disinterest in that body. Instead, a new feeling grew within me—a calm, wonderful sense of peace and relief. My fear of death vanished, replaced by excitement for my new journey. I metaphorically had one foot on Earth and one foot in heaven. And more than anything, I wanted to take another step forward and leave my body behind.

It was not the first bizarre, otherworldly experience I had, though. I had been warned about it. A few months previously, as I sat at my parents' kitchen table putting a thousand-piece puzzle together, I heard a male voice behind my right shoulder.

"You'll be dying soon," it said. "And there's nothing to be afraid of."

I whipped my head around to see who'd spoken. I was alone in the room.

I wasn't sure where the voice came from, but I somehow knew I could trust it. I thought it meant that maybe I'd get into a car accident or something. It seems strange that even though I was only twenty years old, I wasn't terrified by the news of my upcoming death. It seems strange that a disembodied voice was so trustworthy that it shaped my thinking. Because it did, I began mentally preparing for my death and, as I was told, tried not to be afraid.

I didn't tell anyone, especially my husband, Matt, because I couldn't. I didn't want others to think I had lost my mind, hearing voices and anticipating a catastrophe. It never occurred to me that I would die from complications of ulcerative colitis, but it would have made more sense. I had been diagnosed with UC a year before but was still in heavy denial about it. I didn't comprehend that I would never fully recover from a disease that was, in fact, rapidly killing me. I was fine, I told myself, so an auto accident seemed more likely.

Accidents always seemed the likeliest way for young people to die. And I had always been healthy, until age nineteen, when I got heartburn.

This was no ordinary heartburn. This heartburn had superpowers.

It felt like my throat and lungs were on fire, and it went on for days. And into the night. Soon I had to sleep sitting up, and it progressively worsened until I vomited everything I ate.

It was heartburn that felt like the stomach flu. I could not keep any food down. Orange juice felt like drinking fire that burned on the way back up. I swiftly and permanently exiled that from my fridge.

I began running random daily fevers. I felt fine and then my face would sweat like a steamed lobster. The heat traveled through my body, leaving me feeling clammy and freezing, my hair soaking wet. As I got weaker and weaker, Matt took me to and from work because I didn't have the energy to drive. And it got worse. I had a bone-deep exhaustion that never went away.

Matt and I had been married for a little over a year at this point. We met when I was a junior in high school. He was two years older than me and a DJ for a local radio station, which, back then, was the height of cool. He was giving away tickets to a Coolio concert. Coolio, y'all. My gangster, rap-loving heart nearly exploded. It was a match made in heaven—or so I thought. We dated all the way through graduation. Not long after, we got married, bought a house, and started planning our happily ever after. We dreamed of careers, kids, and family holidays in a simple, yet happy, future.

Turns out our pairing was not exactly a fantastic voyage but more like a mildly chaotic road trip with no GPS, a half-flat tire, and someone who kept changing the radio station when my favorite song came on.

This uninvited sickness didn't fit into our future. It wasn't what we planned on when we said, "I do."

I was disappearing, piece by piece, into an illness that consumed my life.

Matt didn't seem to grasp the severity of the storm that had blown into our lives like tumbleweeds settling after the winds die down, prickly and unwanted.

I thought back to the day I received my diagnosis.

After visits with multiple specialists and even more medical tests, with so much blood work I was worried I might run out of blood, my doctor called me into his office.

"Heather, we received the results of your blood work and colonoscopy. You have a chronic condition called severe ulcerative colitis. It's a form of inflammatory bowel disease that causes inflammation, ulcers, and sores in the digestive tract. Ulcerative colitis affects the innermost lining of the large intestine."

I tried to stay composed. Severe ulcerative colitis (because it SUCks).

"Okay . . . so what does this mean? Can I take an antibiotic and it will go away?"

"No, it is lifelong. There will be flare-ups, various symptoms, medications, and possibly surgery. Complications include severe dehydration, a perforated colon, bone loss, and inflammation of the skin, joints, and eyes."

Eyes. What kind of demonic gut disease branched out to mess with the eyes?

I felt the air leave my lungs as I began to understand the gravity of this diagnosis. I was devastated. I wanted to go back to that morning when I was just a normal person without a death sentence hanging over her head.

I don't remember the ride home. I was shell-shocked.

Grief took up residence in my heart.

The next few days were a blur as I cried nonstop. I felt so alone in my struggles. My parents and Matt tried to be supportive when I gave them the news. My mom tried to remain strong, but I could see it in her eyes—the visceral fear, the panic as my health declined. She stood at my stove, making soup from scratch like it was the cure. Her hands trembled slightly as she handed me the steaming bowl. I ate a few bites to appease her, but my appetite was gone. Eating caused so much pain.

Even with her fear of the unknown, she never left me. She was there every minute and for every doctor's appointment. Asking the questions I was too scared to ask. A constant comfort, a shoulder to cry on when the unknown became overwhelming.

Matt, on the other hand, didn't know what to do with me. Ever the optimist, he tried to diffuse the situation with laughter. "Maybe it's not as bad as we think." In his mind, it couldn't possibly be as bad as the doctors made it sound. I was young. I would bounce back. In spite of his positivity, he was overwhelmed, maybe even a little frozen. It was a lot to take in. His wife's health had plummeted swiftly over the last year. He didn't know how to deal with my new companions—grief and pain. Denial felt safer than acknowledging his fears. I didn't blame him. Denial is a great coping strategy—for a while. After all, I could hardly believe it myself.

I read every book I could find on this disease. This was before WebMD was a thing. If it had been available, I would have gone down that rabbit hole as well. The exact cause of ulcerative colitis remains unknown, and there is no cure. This disease usually peaks between the ages of fifteen to thirty and fifty to seventy. Each book and pamphlet offered little hope for a healthy, normal life.

Though I felt relieved that I finally had some answers as to what was causing all of my health problems, I hoped my doctor had misdiagnosed me.

As the disease progressed, it became unresponsive to the multitude of medications my gastroenterologist prescribed. My body was failing fast. It was not okay. It was profoundly, horrifically unfair. I coped with it all using a strategy so brilliant I didn't even realize I'd come up with it: denial.

It was hard work fighting the reality of my diagnosis. But no matter how much pain I was in, I kept my brain in the dark about my gut. My body was providing so much evidence of its own breakdown that my refusal to accept how bad it was could have won me medals. I was aware of the pain; I just wasn't willing to admit the biggest part.

Young and newly married, I should be living the best years of my life. Instead, I was so weak and dehydrated I could not keep any food or fluid in my body. I was still working full-time. Every day, I drank small bottles of Imodium and Pepto Bismol in an attempt to stay hydrated. I went through so many—each a reminder of how much my body struggled to hold on. I would not admit this to myself, but these were actually not the best years of my life.

My doctors tried everything to stabilize my health, but to no avail. I don't know how much of their efforts went to finding a remedy and how much went to finding a way to convince me I was sicker than I wanted to admit. In this, my condition was on my side, not theirs. I could feel myself slipping away, but I was too exhausted and dehydrated to truly understand or admit how bad it was getting. So the denial fed itself in a relentless feedback loop. And the exhaustion fed my denial of the severity. Then I would be so sick I could not think clearly at all. Rinse and repeat. I was eventually forced to quit working. I had always been a hard worker, consistently pulling nine-hour shifts, but in August 1999, I was so weak, all I wanted to do was sleep. But even that was hard to do because my night fevers had me waking up, violently shaking with chills. I could never get past feeling bone-tired. The simplest tasks drained me completely.

And still I denied that anything was really wrong! I pushed myself to be a normal twenty-year-old. Even as I grew worse, I refused to believe it. I couldn't possibly be that sick, I told myself. I did everything I could think of to get better: took all my prescribed medications, did blood work weekly, and even drank a weird dried-herb concoction that smelled and tasted horrible and was supposed to cure me, but each day, I slipped further and further away from health and life.

In October 1999, I woke with bad back pain. My entire back felt like one massive bruise. Breathing was excruciating. Over the next few days, it progressively worsened. I took Tylenol, soaked in hot baths, and used a heating pad, trying to dull the pain. Nothing helped. It became so unbearable I finally asked Mom to take me to the emergency room. Matt was at work, and I didn't think I could wait until he got home.

On the way to the ER, my breathing became so ragged I couldn't take a full breath, and I was getting dizzier by the minute.

Knowing I was going to be admitted, Mom stopped at Target to buy me pajamas since we hadn't brought anything for an overnight stay. I waited in the car while she ran inside. After a few minutes, things got worse. I needed to get to the hospital. Feeling like I would suffocate before she came out of the store, I considered crawling into the store to find her, but I didn't have the strength to get out of the car. When my mom finally returned, every breath felt like fire scorching my lungs, and I could barely find the strength to move.

When we arrived at the emergency room, a nurse put me in a

wheelchair and took me straight to the front of the line so I could be admitted. As the nurse wheeled me to the elevator, I was still fighting with my emotions. I was relieved to be where I could get some oxygen, but a pit of dread had formed in my stomach. I didn't know what was coming, but I knew it was bad.

After the blood work and a colonoscopy with biopsies, I learned I had pneumonia and that my lungs had collapsed, both complications of the ulcerative colitis.

It took four days of hospitalization until I was stable enough to be released. They said I had failed to achieve recovery with sulfasalazine and Dipentum. I was sent home with a prescription for 6-mercaptop-urine, a chemotherapy drug generally used to treat leukemia, to be used in conjunction with prednisone and Asacol HD, that I was already taking. "I won. I cheated death, and that voice was wrong . . . lucky me!"

Chapter 2

I'll Be Home for Christmas —Unless Admitted Again

T wo months later, on December 15, I was back in the ER. My dad drove me this time as Matt was once again at work. I'd been experiencing persistent high fevers, along with nausea and dizziness.

Following another physical exam and some lab work, I was diagnosed with probable viral syndrome and then sent home with instructions to schedule an appointment with my gastroenterologist, whom I had been in constant contact with. He had suggested surgery, so I was not too keen on seeing him again, but I dutifully made the appointment. The ER doctor told me if the fevers did not go down (or stop) and I couldn't tolerate my medications, I would be admitted the next time I came in.

Five days later, on December 20, I was back at the ER running a fever of 104.4. For most of December, I battled high fevers nothing could touch. Despite shaking uncontrollably from the cold, the heat inside me wouldn't let up. The fevers left my clothes soaking wet to the point where I was changing outfits four to five times a day and multiple times during the night. When I talked, my teeth chattered. I popped Tylenol every four hours, wore shirts under heavy sweaters and leggings, and wrapped myself in blankets to stay warm. When that didn't work, I took steaming-hot baths in an effort to get my burning body to *feel* warm.

There was another detail about this next stretch of hospital stays: I could not sit down. I frequently passed out, as one does when starving and dying.

Before one ER trip, I passed out somewhere near the top of the stairs at my house. I clutched the railing, my breathing shallow and fast. My vision started to swim, and the world tilted.

"Not again," I whispered.

And then I crashed down the stairs like a rag doll, limbs tangled, body coming to a stop with a sickening thump on the cold, hard tile.

When I came to, I lay sprawled upside down on the bottom step.

For a minute, I lost my breath.

My first thought was, *Did I just break my butt?*

Pain screamed through my back and tailbone like they were on fire.

Yup, I'd broken my butt. I'd definitely broken my butt.

I dragged myself down the hall inch by inch, like a war casualty, every movement feeling like hot coals beneath my tailbone.

I whimpered and then laughed. *This is ridiculous*, I thought. Chronic illness, fainting, and now a broken butt?

I vowed to never sit until it healed. The pain was too intense.

I was smart enough to know I needed a miracle. The medication was obviously not bringing me into remission like my doctors hoped it would.

Now, I found myself in the ER again, where the attending ER physician assigned to my care examined me and then ordered more blood work and abdominal X-rays. He worried that I was not responding to outpatient therapy and about how I had come back to the ER so often. (He was right; I visited the ER so often I should have gotten a punch card for a free stay.) He wanted to pinpoint why I was not responding to any of my medications. Since October, each time I tapered off my high doses of prednisone, my body suffered a severe relapse of ulcerative colitis.

The doctor decided to admit me so I could be stabilized. He ordered an abdominal CT scan and fluids to help with my dehydration and immobility while we awaited answers from imaging and blood work.

I was dozing in that half-conscious state of in between where I wasn't sure if things were *real* real or dream real.

And I had a vision. It wasn't of heaven or the future. It was of Fabio. My brain was not being normal. I decided to go with it.

Fabio, long blond hair blowing around his face and shoulders, came right into my hospital room, backlit by the glaring lights of the hallway. I may have heard a whisper of soft Italian music. Or it could have been the blood pressure cuff sighing as it released? Who wouldn't sigh for Fabio? True, he wore scrubs and a stethoscope. His face was thoughtful as he sat down on the edge of my bed.

His blue eyes seeing right into my heart, he said those magical words: "We need to remove your large intestine."

Total buzzkill.

In my foggy brain, I wondered when Fabio had gone to medical school. He continued to speak, though his English was much more articulate than in his 1980s shampoo commercials.

"In order to save your life . . . The operation is common, but drastic. It will excise an entire organ. We divert one end of your intestine, which is part of the bowel, through a new opening we'll create in your stomach. This stomach hole, called a stoma, will allow your small intestine to send waste to a colostomy bag, which collects it"—Fabio blinked as he finished—"outside the body."

I didn't blink back. I was in denial again, which was better than admitting I was in a hospital room.

I said, "Can I go home for my family Christmas party first? Then, as soon as I check back in, we can do this, uh, thing you're talking about."

Fabio and my dad exchanged a meaningful glance. "Heather," the doctor spoke a little more slowly this time, "your large intestine has become so infected and inflamed and so riddled with ulcers that unless we take it out, you will die within twenty-four hours."

Denial is a harsh mistress. "I can make it back before then, I think," I said.

Fabio's gorgeous hair seemed to wither a little as his shoulders slumped. I could tell he was frustrated, but so was I. He said, "Do you not understand that we are about to order an operating room to be prepped right *now*? This procedure has to happen immediately. So I am sorry, but, no, you can't leave the hospital. I am sure your family will miss you at the party, but it is better than missing you at every Christmas from now on."

Those words sank in.

And, finally, I let the fear in—fear of death, but also of paralysis during the surgery, of waking up and feeling the cutting but unable to move. I was afraid for real. I wasn't sitting in my regular doctor's office, talking over him, shutting him down with waves of cheery, chattery denial as he urged me to consider this very surgery several times over the past week—before it became this severe.

I weighed ninety-four pounds, having lived on rice baby cereal, broth, and applesauce for weeks. I couldn't keep food in my body. I was so severely dehydrated, weak, and malnourished I randomly passed out throughout the day and woke with blocks of memory gone —and now a broken butt.

Dr. Fabio left the room to let us speak with Dr. Briggs, who would perform the operation. As he walked in, I watched him intently. He would make the first cut—the cut that would forever draw a line between before and after. He carried himself with a quiet intensity. He was reserved—not cold, but calm and focused in a way that made you pay attention. His voice soft and deliberate, he chose his words carefully, letting each syllable land with an understanding of what lay ahead.

He grabbed a piece of paper to diagram what would happen to my body during surgery. Blue ink swirled across the white space. My shell of protective pretense and denial began to crack. In that hospital room, I had one last, desperate thought that if I pretended I wasn't sick, I would be okay and could go back home. I didn't want to talk about it or think about it. I wanted to resume the life I had when I was healthy. The reality, however, was that I was so sick I was, in fact, dying. My throat tightened. I struggled to hold back the tears. They came anyway, wildly, uninvited. I felt it fully now, more afraid than ever. My life was about to change forever.

I thought back to when I quit my job the previous August. Ever since, I had failed to maintain any remission from UC whatsoever, even on huge doses of heavy-duty medication. I took my sixty milligrams of steroids every day for thirteen months and, as mentioned, could not taper off them without spiraling into serious relapse. Though the steroid side effects were bad, they were the lesser of two evils. Whenever I tried to taper, it felt like I had been beaten with a baseball bat. Showers felt like millions of nails being hammered into my skin. My least favorite side effect was moon face. A friend helpfully nicknamed me Chipmunk. My favorite side effect was the energy. I had my house so organized that even the cereal boxes in my food pantry were in order from tallest to shortest.

As I lay in my hospital bed after talking with the surgeon, that energy was gone. I felt small, defeated, and deflated—like a kid's balloon that's been popped—and knew it would get worse. I closed my eyes and zoned out as my parents, Matt, and the medical team discussed the pros and cons of the surgery. The fight had left me. I didn't want to be part of the conversation. I would have the surgery because there was no other option.

Scheduled for December 23, 1999, the surgery would consist of a colectomy and an ileo-anal pull through (IPPA), which basically meant the removal of my entire colon, rectum, and appendix so that all the infection was removed from my system. The plan was that I would spend a few days in hospital recovery after surgery and then be released with a colostomy bag while I healed. Once I was stronger, I would return for two more surgeries, with the final surgery being the construction of a J-pouch, which would replace the parts they removed. The surgeon would construct it from the ileum, which is the end of the small intestine. This pouch is sewn into the shape of a J, hence the name.

The J-pouch would give me the freedom to live a more normal life, and the plan sounded good because I would be alive. I worried about how much my body would change with all the scarring from so many surgeries. Then again, if I died, any scars wouldn't matter.

As I lay in my hospital room, preparing for surgery and trying to breathe through the rising panic, the door swung open, and there they were—my three brothers, Josh, Jeremy, and Shawn.

Josh came in first, cool and collected, with that chill energy he always carried. Still in high school, like Jeremy, he spent his time going to concerts, hanging out with friends, and just being a teenager. Today, his face was serious.

Jeremy followed. He was rough around the edges and always fidgeting with something in his hands, like he was halfway through fixing an engine or machine. His quiet personality shone through as he stood in the corner against the wall.

And then there was Shawn, technically not my brother by blood but in every way that mattered. He and Jeremy had been best friends since childhood. During our teen years, Shawn came and then simply never left. My parents became his parents. He became part of us, an honorary sibling, the brother I never knew I needed. A year older than me, he was fiercely loyal. I couldn't imagine life without my three brothers. We were tight.

Their presence that day calmed the rising panic and fears that haunted my waking moments. I had been spiraling with worst-case scenarios, but for that brief window in time, surrounded by my family, I felt anchored. I wasn't alone in the upcoming storm.

December 23 arrived, and I was prepped for the surgery. I felt miserable. Physically, I hurt all over. Emotionally, I was exhausted. And despite that long-ago reassurance of the invisible kitchen voice, I worried about dying. Terrified of what I was about to undergo, my tears flowed freely as the nurses wheeled me into surgery. *I guess I won't make it to my family Christmas party*, I thought grimly.

The bright lights of the operating room were jarring, and it was so cold. Operating rooms are kept cold to help with sterilization, but that also makes them feel like meat lockers.

I couldn't take full breaths because I was crying and shaking. My efforts to calm down were not working. I wanted to be anywhere but here. I had never had surgery—and this was a major one, with countless risks due to my weakened, malnourished state and the sheer magnitude of having so much of my insides removed.

As the anesthesia took hold, a wave of relief washed over me, loosening the tension that gripped my body for days. My nurse gently told me to count backward. My sobs subsided, and I slowly surrendered—drifting into the darkness.

I woke up groggy but in intense pain, surprised I had made it through. I could hear the beeping of the machines around me along with the conversations of the people in the room.

I could feel someone standing next to me, but I was afraid to open my eyes. When I finally did, a nurse smiled down at me.

"How are you feeling?" she asked, her voice soft, distant.

I wanted to answer, but the words got stuck somewhere inside me. *Cold.*

Shaky.

Everything inside me trembled—my body, my thoughts, my grip on reality. "Do you have a heated blanket?" I replied. As she covered me in the blanket that had just come out of the warmer, my body relaxed a little. Then I felt the burning in my incision. When I remembered why I was here, a tear slid down my cheek. I tried to move my hand toward my stomach to check for the bandages. She took my hand in hers and explained that I was in the recovery room and I had been a trooper during surgery. Everything had gone according to plan, with no complications. She was going to keep me here to monitor my vitals and pain levels. She had a calming voice, and I felt safe with her.

When I was transferred to my room a few hours later, I finally got a chance to look at my eight-inch incision, which had been stapled closed. It looked red and angry, as if an incision could have an emotion. And, as promised, a colostomy bag hung outside my stomach. It filled with waste anytime I ate. I was mortified. My body looked so weird, so foreign. I didn't want anyone to see me like this. I made sure my hospital gown and blanket covered as much as possible, at all times—my armor against the world. It was humiliating to have to wear a clear bag full of waste on the outside of my body. I felt self-conscious, exposed, and deeply vulnerable. The stitches that were supposed to dissolve itched mercilessly. (Incidentally, not all of them dissolved. Ten years later—yes, a full decade—late at night, I took a scalpel, scissors, and a pair of tweezers, like I was auditioning for a back-alley surgery scene, and cut a small slice in my abdomen. Voilà! I pulled out a three-inch-long blue thread that had started poking through my skin like it wanted out. It was a process because it had grown into some of the muscle. Eww, I know. But I was impressed with my handiwork.)

To help me prepare for discharge, I was assigned a special nurse who taught me how to care for and change the bag to be self-sufficient. She tried to be gentle when she removed the sticky tape used to attach it to my body, but my skin was so thin and fragile that when she pulled the tape off, layers of skin peeled away.

"Ouch!" I gasped, the pain sharp and immediate—each time stealing my breath before I could catch it. She covered me with a rough hospital blanket, trying to stop my shivering. She was a kind, patient, grandmotherly type who tried to comfort me as she worked.

"You will not have this bag forever. You can and will live a very fulfilled and healthy life," she said. I wanted to believe her, but in those moments, all I felt was raw hurt and shame.

She told stories of other patients who lived with colostomy bags—people who had healed, recovered, and gone on to live full lives.

One day, I was in the middle of a full-blown pity party when she walked in.

"I have someone I want you to meet," she said, eyes twinkling.

Another patient on my floor was recovering from a similar surgery but was in worse condition than I was. He had a family of his own and had been sick for a long time—longer than me.

When he walked the hall for his daily rounds, she had him stop by my room to introduce himself. He leaned against the doorframe, holding his IV pole, his breathing labored. He gave me a tired smile.

"Do you regret having the surgery?" I blurted after he introduced himself. I was not convinced I could live like this, even for a few months. They told me the colostomy bag was only temporary—just until my body had time to heal—but that didn't make it any easier to accept. I was desperate for some truth, not some sugar-coated lie. I needed it straight from someone who had walked the path I now walked, someone facing the same horror and humiliation I did.

I expected him to say the surgery was a big mistake, like I felt mine had been.

What he said next surprised me.

His surgery, although painful, would give him the chance to watch his children grow up. Without it, he would only be a picture in a photo album and a memory. He could now be at his kids' high school and college graduations. He would be there to dance at their weddings. He would welcome his grandbabies into the world. He would celebrate anniversaries with his beloved wife.

This perspective was one I had not thought about as I wallowed in my misery. I thanked him as he left to go back to his room.

Whenever my nurse visited after this, I asked for updates on my newfound friend.

Later, when I was transferred to another floor, my friend and I lost touch. I do hope he's lived a long, full life and achieved everything he wanted to.

When I was alone, I spent a lot of time looking at my abdomen, wondering how my life had so quickly changed from that of a normal girl to that of one who was so sickly she had to ring the nurses' bell for help standing up. I am an independent person who resented not being able to take care of myself. I didn't want to look, or be, weak. I felt like some of the nurses looked through me and didn't see me as a person, just a very sick individual they were required to care for. Each time a new nurse came to check my vitals and incision, they glanced at my medical chart before looking at me. As they read through the notes, looks of pity crossed their faces. "You're a very sick girl," I heard most often when they finally took a look at their patient. I knew this. I lived with the reality every single day. I didn't need to be reminded.

I wanted to scream at them. "Don't talk down to me like I won't understand what you are saying. I'm sick, not stupid. Don't give medical updates to my family while acting like I am not in the room. I want a say in my care!"

I wanted this to be over with. I wanted to get the sleep I needed for my body to heal, but nurses were in and out of my room, constantly checking my vitals. I wished I could lock my door and block them from entering with their needles and test orders. More than anything, I wished I were home—in my own soft bed, wrapped in my favorite pink, floral blanket, the one that always lulled me to sleep at night. I missed the way the sun shone through my bedroom window in the early morning hours, waking me from a deep slumber and warming my cheeks.

I missed being well enough to go to dinner on Friday night with Matt and our friends. Instead, I tried to be the model patient who did what I was told as I felt parts of my former self slipping away. I felt broken and didn't recognize the person staring back at me in the mirror. Worst of all, I was forgetting what it felt like to be a normal twenty-year-old. I felt much older. I felt resigned to accept that my life might never be happy again.

I spent Christmas 1999 in a hospital room recovering from surgery. The only memory I have of Christmas Day was of my family bringing a few of my gifts for me to open. I was embarrassed that I hadn't had time to get everyone gifts. They tried to make it a happy day despite the strange and sterile setting. It was as if they were trying a little too hard—filling the room with noise and discomfort none of us wanted to name.

I didn't really feel like interacting with anyone. My body felt like it had been stitched together by fire. My nurse must have known this because she kept pushing the button on my morphine pump which, while it didn't do much for the pain, did keep me in a hazy and dreamlike state, detached from reality. The room was blurry and spinning; everyone swayed around like sea creatures at high tide. I will never understand using morphine as a recreational drug since I hate the way it affects me. I was pretty out of it, sleeping on and off.

Chapter 3

Party Like It's 1999—And Leave Your Body Doing It

The first time I noticed that something felt off was New Year's Eve 1999, as I was still recovering in the hospital.

It was Y2K. No one knew what could happen to computers and other digital equipment when the clock struck midnight. Though it seems minor in retrospect, this was a real concern. My doctors and nurses were worried that the machines and computers keeping me and the other patients alive might shut down. There were generators on-site, but no one knew how bad it might get if the computers and medical equipment failed.

Matt, Mom, and my brothers Jeremy and Shawn were by my side at the hospital, ready in case everything spiraled into chaos. We had the television on, watching the countdown to the New Year as well as coverage from all over the world as the new year, century, and millennium swept in. We watched it happen in Australia and saw the ball drop in New York.

And the chaos did not come. When the clock struck midnight in Salt Lake City, Utah, nothing happened to any of the computers or medical equipment at the hospital. I felt bad for everyone who'd charged up their credit cards, thinking they would be wiped clean in the new year if the computers crashed and lost all their data. They still had to pay their bills into the new millennium.

I had other things to think about.

This was the night I began leaving my body.

That evening, as two nurses came to check my vitals and examine my incision, I felt myself lift off the bed and float upward. I rose until I was level with their shoulders as they stood on either side of me. Though I still lay down—completely vertical—my body levitated effortlessly, the sensation surreal.

But no one seemed to notice. I wondered why no one was alarmed like I was. This was so confusing! I didn't say anything because it did not make sense and I knew levitating was not normal.

No one else in the room seemed confused. No one said, "Hey, there, Heather, why are you floating three feet above your bed?"

So I decided not to draw attention to myself. After the nurses left, I gently floated back down onto the bed and finished watching the New Year's celebrations with my family. Then I went to sleep for the night.

Chapter 4

Spillin' My Guts

On January 3, Dr. Briggs came to do his morning rounds around 6 a.m.

Breakfast had been delivered to my room, and I had been given a piece of toast. You have no idea how happy I was to see that piece of toast.

I had been on total parenteral nutrition, with a feeding tube up my nose and down into my stomach. Oh, how I missed chewing and tasting the different textures of food. And here was toast! Simple, glorious toast.

Right before I took a bite, Dr. Briggs ripped the toast from my hand.

"Is your mom at work?" he asked over my cry of dismay.

He walked over to look out the window with his arms crossed over his chest. I was so distraught that he had taken away my toast that all I could think about was how good that first crunchy, buttery, warm bite was going to taste. I tried to stop myself from crying.

"Why'd you take my food?"

He came back to my bedside. "You've had what we call a small bowel evisceration."

I snuck a peek at my abdomen. Sure enough, something pink and sort of streaked with blood was bunched up inside the colostomy bag. I suspected my intestine. And my blood.

I was not going to get my toast back.

I felt so defeated.

I would have to endure another surgery. I hated the disorienting feeling of coming out of anesthesia and the idea of yet another scar. My doctor called my mother and asked her to come to the hospital immediately. She worked nearby and could be there within five minutes.

Throughout my hospitalization, whenever there was an emergency, my doctor called Mom, not Matt. She was more responsive. She dropped everything and rushed to the hospital without hesitation. Matt was overwhelmed by the intensity of my medical needs, and as the primary breadwinner at just twenty-two years old was often consumed with work. He didn't always know how to navigate the crisis we were living through. Still, I knew he cared—he was just coping the only way he knew how. And thankfully, I had other family members there to comfort me when he couldn't.

While we waited for Mom, I got stress doses of prednisone. Once she arrived and came to my room to squeeze my hand and look brave and say goodbye, I was wheeled down the hall to a surgery room, with Mom and a few nurses watching from the sidelines like some weird farewell party.

I found myself back in the cold, brightly lit surgery room, and sadness engulfed me.

This was a large setback. I would have to stay in the hospital even longer while I recovered. The J-pouch had detached and emerged from my stomach. This was bad news since it was supposed to take the place of my colostomy bag during the final reversal surgery. If the pouch became damaged and unworkable, I might have a colostomy bag forever. To help minimize the number of daily pokes I needed for IV meds and labs, a nurse placed a central line in one of my larger veins during this surgery.

The surgery went as well as could be expected and was considered a success. And I was once again sent to the recovery ward for the nurses to monitor me until I came out of my anesthesia haze.

Over the next few days, I slept on and off, covered in heated hospital blankets as I tried to get strong enough to go home.

My best friend, Breezi, worked nearby and came after work to keep me entertained and take my mind off the daily reminders of my new life.

We first met at the job I had been forced to quit when I became sick.

On that fateful day of our first meeting, I was eating lunch in the break room. A girl in hospital scrubs walked in with what can only be described as a gangster stroll. She looked like she owned the place. She looked angry and, truth be told, a little scary. *I hope she is not the new girl*, I thought to myself. I was sure she would beat me in an arm wrestle. She sat down and introduced herself, and I realized pretty quickly that her tough exterior housed someone with the gentlest heart. We became fast friends.

Each day, we shared lunch at the hospital cafeteria across from our medical office. She gave me the tomatoes from her sandwich. I gave her my lunch meat. We were the perfect pair—a vegetarian and a carnivore. She became my person—my protector and closest friend. We spent hours on the phone at night, shopped on weekends, and lunched at Olive Garden and Sizzler. We were both eighteen years old with our entire lives ahead of us.

Having Breezi at the hospital turned a really scary situation into a bearable one. Like girls at a sleepover, we laughed and gossiped about co-workers and patients back at her job. We daydreamed about the things we'd do after I was healthy again. Maybe a road trip with all our favorite snacks.

In these moments, I could leave behind the awful sounds and scents of the hospital and pretend we were having a girl's day out at the mall.

I know it was hard for Breezi to be there as often as she was while working full-time and balancing all her responsibilities. But she never complained. She showed up for me again and again, giving me a safe space to express my fears, her comfort and love aiding my recovery.

Chapter 5

Watching Myself While Out of My Body

On January 11, while I was still recovering inpatient, I experienced a second, small bowel evisceration. Once again, it was emergency surgery to return my small intestine to where it belonged.

After surgery, I was transferred to the med-surg/ICU unit on the sixth floor.

In my already weakened state, this surgery took an even heavier toll on me. I spiraled downward swiftly. It was my third major operation in just two weeks, my body robbed of the time it desperately needed to heal from the first two.

My parents were with me until 7:00 p.m., when visiting hours ended. Dad shared with me that an entry in his journal for that night said, "She is not in good shape, but she is still alive."

My parents came to the hospital around 9:00 a.m. the next day. I glanced over and heard my mom gasp. I knew I didn't look good, but her face told me how bad it was. "I'm going to clear out Heather's old hospital room," I heard my mom whisper to my dad. She avoided eye contact with me and looked like she would cry.

She was terrified I was going to die. No matter how many times she said, "You're going to get through this," I saw the unspoken doubt. Every beep of the monitor made her flinch.

I was her child, and she was watching that child disappear. The helplessness was unbearable for her.

Every day, though, she showed up with every ounce of her courage. She stood between me and the darkness—fiercely loving me. But she was breaking. I could see it when she let her guard down when she didn't think I was watching.

At 10:00 a.m., as my dad watched the critical care team work on me, I heard him say "Yes?" as he looked at the nurses and then scanned the room. He later shared with me what happened.

Your mom and I walked into your room. There were eight nurses in the room. They were moving quickly, prepping tubes, medications, and machines. You were lying on the bed and looked near death. Your fever was high, and your face was bright red. Your chest was rising and falling unevenly. The air in the room was filled with tension. Your mom left to gather your belongings from your previous room. It was just the nurses, you, and me.

Then I heard a gentle female voice, clear as a bell. 'Craig.'

'Yes,' I answered.

The nurses didn't respond. They were focused on your care. They were new to your team, they didn't know my name, and your mom wasn't in the room to have said my name. I was confused where the voice had come from. I waited for a response but did not receive one.

He told me that when no one answered him, he realized someone had said his name and that it was someone in the room who could not be seen.

This was the first time the Other Side presented to my family, perhaps to provide comfort or let them know of their concern and understanding of the coming trials. This voice did not scare my dad, although he did wonder who it belonged to. "Maybe it was my mother, who passed away a year before," he suggested.

My dad wrote in his journal that night that I looked worse than the night before.

I was extremely critical at this point. I had aspirated into my lungs and developed acute respiratory distress syndrome (ARDS), a life-threatening condition that allows fluid to leak into the lungs. I also had perihilar pulmonary edema, another serious lung complication. Whatever their formal names, these conditions made every breath difficult, painful, and frightening. My cells couldn't get oxygen.

Oxygen and blood circulation are important for all body functions, including healing injuries and illnesses. Because my body was so badly worn down, I was also becoming septic. They used to call sepsis "blood poisoning," but it's more complicated than that. Sepsis occurs when chemicals released in the bloodstream to fight infection trigger inflammation throughout the body. This can cause changes that damage the organs, causing them to fail, sometimes even resulting in death. Complicated intra-abdominal infections are the second most common cause of septic death in the intensive care unit. I was unlucky enough to add that to my list of complications.

But wait. There's more.

I also developed tachycardia, a condition where the heart rate exceeds one hundred beats per minute while at rest. For a healthy adult, a normal resting heart rate ranges between sixty and one hundred beats per minute. Mine spiked as high as 190. My body was so weak that every breath demanded all my strength—both mental and physical. I was so exhausted I wasn't sure how much longer I could keep going.

My heart felt like it was going to explode out of my chest, the beating so loud I was sure everyone else could hear it. I was terrified. I could tell that the critical care nurses and doctors were equally worried. I tried to tell my family how scared I was, but I couldn't form coherent sentences. It felt like the air was rapidly being sucked in and out of my lungs with a vacuum. Though all my effort went into trying to control my breathing, I could not force it to slow to a normal rate. I hoped that if I could get control of it, I wouldn't have to be intubated.

My mom sat next to me on my bed, clearly worried. She placed my hand in hers. Her cold hands trembled. Her eyes were bloodshot from crying. She looked gaunt and pale. When she tried to soothe my worries, her voice broke, layered with grief. "I know you are scared. I am too. I am here with you. I'm not leaving you," Mom repeated over and over as I gasped for air.

Her fear made it harder for me to breathe because my fear of dying was getting worse each time I took a shaky half breath. I felt like I was losing control, which terrified me.

"Why can't anyone help me?" I cried out.

I was given three pints of blood, with five to eight critical care nurses in the room at all times working tirelessly to stabilize me. As the room grew more chaotic and crowded, my family was asked to step outside. My healthcare team made the decision to intubate me.

My parents had met up with my mother- and father-in-law in the waiting room down the hall when a doctor and nurse came and told them they could come back in. Matt was called at work and told he needed to come to the hospital.

As our parents started to walk toward my room, a group of six nurses came running down the hall, pushing a patient in a hospital bed. The patient had a breathing mask over her face, and the nurses manually pumped air to help her breathe. One of them yelled, "Get out of the way!" as they ran past my family.

As soon as my family realized it was me, my dad and father-in-law went to ask the nurses what happened. My mom, who thought I was dead, refused to go with them. My mother-in-law said it was the worst thing she had ever seen. The nurses told them I was fine and being transported to the trauma unit for extra care.

I was not fine.

My body was not fine. But I might have been. Because it was at this time that I found myself watching with a strange, distant curiosity as the nurses frantically worked to stabilize that body in the hospital bed. I sat off to the side in a small area with three rows of concrete seats arranged in a half circle—like stadium seats at an outdoor venue. The scene felt surreal, as if I watched the drama of someone else's life unfolding before me. A nurses' station sat directly to my right, where a few nurses did paperwork and answered phones. One held a clipboard with a pencil swinging from it by a string as she walked.

The hospital bed was about one hundred feet in front of me, and the scene was total chaos. Though I didn't know her, I felt sorry for the young girl they were trying to save. I watched for a few minutes as the staff held her down to insert a tube into her throat. She resisted every step of the way, hysterical and shaking and breathing heavily. Fear radiated from her like buzzing, broken energy, her eyes wide and wild. I felt sorry for this suffering person, but I really didn't have any other thoughts besides a mild interest in the scene. It was like watching a movie and having empathy for the character, but not enough to become emotionally attached. I could feel all the emotions and thoughts of the nurses, too, as they worked on the girl. They thought she was not going to make it, and they were scared. I didn't know how it was possible to understand their thoughts, yet I could.

I had no emotional connection, no sense of ownership or recognition, of the body in that bed. It was only after several minutes of watching—just observing from a distance—that the truth slowly dawned on me: the frightened girl they were trying so desperately to save was me. I was stunned. How could it be? And yet it was. What struck me even more was the absence of something that had defined my every waking moment: pain. I had been in agony for so long I could hardly remember what it felt like not to hurt—and suddenly it was gone. The weight of suffering had lifted, and in its place was silence, stillness.

No one noticed or acknowledged me sitting and watching. But I felt safe. Most importantly, I did not feel the searing pain in my incision, which always felt like someone had stuck a sharp knife in a fire and then sliced my abdomen open with it. My tailbone wasn't sore, I wasn't struggling to breathe, and I felt lighter than I could ever remember.

I felt happier and healthier than I had my entire life. I was content to stay where I was and watch all the commotion around me. My emotions were different than usual in that I did not feel any worry over an outcome. I was detached, but felt a serene peace I had never experienced. I also had absolutely no desire to return to my body. I would have been fine to stay where I was forever. It felt like time didn't exist. I enjoyed watching the rhythm of everyone working together for a common goal. The entire area was filled with a glowing yellowish-white foggy light that felt gently comforting and warm. I could not see anything beyond this light and didn't think to question how I could watch my body while also being outside of it.

I continued to watch the nurses working on me until I was intubated, sedated, and stabilized. My body was then transferred back to the shock-trauma ICU, where I remained sedated and slept through the rest of the night.

At some point, I must have popped back into my body because I no longer watched the scene and have no further memory of it.

My heart and lung doctor, Dr. Pearce, noted in his consultation report: "Critically ill with severe respiratory failure at this time and hopefully an etiology can be found and repaired quickly." He also noted that he would continue to assist with critical care management. A chest X-ray taken on this same day found that when I was intubated, they'd placed the tube six centimeters too far into my lung. This is called "bronchus intubation," and it can cause all kinds of complications. The findings were phoned into the med-surg unit, and I have to assume the situation was corrected immediately. I do wonder if this mistake contributed to my situation becoming even more critical than it might have been otherwise.

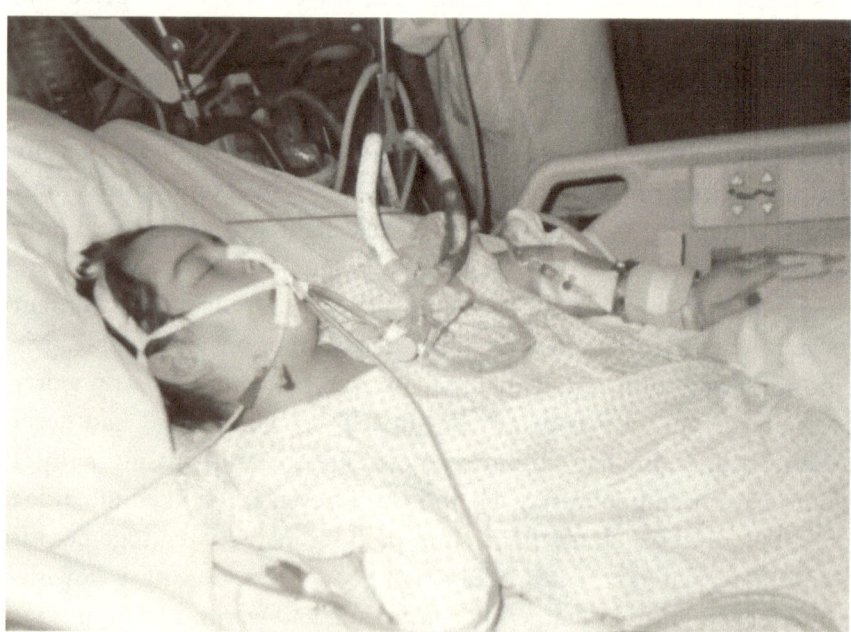

Chapter 6

I Was Literally Beside Myself

Sometime late in the night on January 12, I awoke, back in my body. My room was pitch-black, and I felt something huge and horrible in my mouth, like a big, chewy, plastic straw. I couldn't fully close my mouth around it, and I hated it.

I tried to bring my hand up to my mouth to see what it was.

"Stop that! Put your hands down! Don't touch your face!"

There was a person with me here in the dark!

A man I did not recognize sat in a chair next to my bed; it seemed his job was to terrify me.

When I startled, he doubled down again. "Heather, stop! Do *not* touch your face!"

My body felt heavy with exhaustion, and I was still woozy from the anesthesia. My fever hovered around 104.4, so I also had wet cloths on my head and a box fan to try to control it. I fell asleep but woke up again and again.

This man, who I later learned was named Harlan, was my nurse. He tied my hands to the side rails of the bed so I could not pull out my tube. All night long I would wake up disoriented. Nurse Harlan would chastise me, and then I would fall asleep again. Harlan was abusive throughout my stay in shock trauma. I was supposed to have my body repositioned every few hours to prevent bedsores. Most nurses were gentle about it. Not Harlan. He pulled me across the bed by my ankles to sit me up when my time to walk the hallway arrived each day. This opened up the painful bedsores that had formed on my back, which caused bleeding and a horrific burning sensation.

These cycles were among the most traumatizing of my entire ordeal. I could not speak with the awful intubation, and I was too drugged to write anything. Even if I had been able to, it was too dark in the room. I felt lethargic, feverish, drugged, and confused, all compounded by the yelling of Harlan the Horrible.

I found a way to fight back.

The room was quiet except for the soft whoosh of the ventilator and the occasional beep of the monitor. I lay in bed, pale and in pain, but my eyes were alert. Mom and Breezi quietly hovered around my bed.

Harlan the Horrible walked in, shattering the calm.

It was go time! I grabbed my notepad from my tray and, with tremendous effort, scribbled furiously despite my shaky hands. It took a minute, but I finally slapped the page face-up on my chest, like a battle flag.

In huge, barely legible lettering, I had written "ASSHOLE." If I'd had the strength, I would have underlined the word twice, then written, "Go to hell!"

I pointed at Harlan and flipped him off.

"Heather!" Mom shrieked after gasping loud enough to wake a coma patient. I was afraid she would snatch my paper away. She looked embarrassed. She probably wouldn't be hanging my artwork on her fridge anytime soon. It was a shame, really.

My sweet, very devout Mormon mom who never uttered a swear word assured Harlan, "She didn't mean it."

Wait, what? Who's side was she on? I glared at her.

Breezi read the paper, just as quick to jump in and save me. "Oh yeah. Yes, she does mean it!" It was the clearest communication I'd had in days. She *got* me.

Breezi cackled with laughter. I wanted to laugh with her, but my abdomen and everything else hurt too much. Breezi knew me well enough to know I wouldn't have written that unless there was a valid reason. Always my protector, she shot daggers at Harlan. I wanted her to challenge him to a duel.

Harlan, not used to being confronted, opened and closed his mouth without saying anything. He looked timid and surprised. He scurried out of the room like the vile rat he was, leaving behind the faint smell of latex gloves and sweat. The door clicked shut.

I wanted them to know how mean he was, but my communication skills were so limited.

I wanted to tell them Harlan was a monster and I meant what I said and more! I wanted them to know I trembled every time I heard his voice. I daydreamed of being strong enough to surprise him by punching him in the face the next time he hurt me. None of these words were available to me at that moment, but as always, Breezi had my back.

Later, when I could speak again and I told my mom in brutal detail how awful Harlan had been, her face darkened with rage.

"How *dare* he treat you that way. I want to kill him," she seethed.

Her voice trembled with fury—protective, raw, and fierce. I was her only daughter, and no one had the right to hurt me. Her love wrapped around me like armor, even in my most broken moments.

I still can't understand how a grown man who is supposed to help patients could be so cruel to someone so fragile. Except for the obvious —he was an asshole.

During this part of my hospitalization in the shock trauma unit, my room was directly across from the nurses' station and—somehow —next door to the wife of Thomas S. Monson, who would later become the president of The Church of Jesus Christ of Latter-day Saints. She had fallen on the ice and broken a hip.

Thomas Monson had a special room for him and his security detail so he didn't have to wait in the regular family waiting room. But even with that all going on, he took the time to visit with my parents.

At the time, my family was active in the LDS religion, and his visits brought them a deep sense of comfort. They shared stories and offered prayers—for his wife, for me, for our healing—their voices weaving hope into the stillness of those hospital days.

Although I was raised in the faith, my pioneer ancestors having walked across the frozen plains with handcarts to reach Utah, I had always felt like an outsider looking in. Something about it never quite fit for me, even as a small child. I found myself going through the motions, trying to convince myself that this was my path in life. But deep down, I always felt like I was pretending.

I kept those thoughts to myself, smiling, nodding, and trying to make it feel real.

Lying in a hospital bed, stripped of everything familiar—dignity, privacy, and even a sense of self—I began to see with a clarity I'd never known before. I began to experience something raw and sacred, beyond the borders of religion. I began to discover a different kind of spirituality, one that felt deeply personal and familiar, one that didn't require a building or label.

Watching my parents find comfort in their prayers with President Monson, I didn't feel disconnected or judgmental. I felt grateful. Their faith was real to them. But I also knew with certainty that my path would lead somewhere else, somewhere that felt more like home to my soul.

I didn't feel lost; I felt led.

In the hospital, it was common to hear the loudspeaker announcing a code-blue medical emergency with another critical-care patient and to see flashing lights above the doors of the hospital rooms as the nurses were called to help. Quite often, I saw the flashing lights of the Life Flight helicopter as it landed nearby. I did not get much sleep because of the constant vigilance of the nurses who were in my room more often than they were not.

I stayed in shock trauma until January 14, when my doctors felt I was stable enough to be transferred to the respiratory special care unit.

Chapter 7

Diving into Timeless Knowledge

The entire time I was hospitalized, I had a morphine pump to control my pain, but I refused to push it. I hated the way the morphine made me feel. Whenever the nurses pushed the pump, it felt like my eyes rolled around in the back of my head and my tongue curled up, swollen in my mouth. It also made it hard to communicate. I felt like I had no control over what happened to me. As it turns out, I didn't just dislike the pump, I was having allergic reactions to the morphine, hence the swollen tongue, along with rashes all over my body, whenever they dosed me.

From the second week of January almost until I was discharged, my soul wasn't always inside my body. Whenever the pain became too much, I popped out, just like when I watched my nurses ventilate me. I could leave effortlessly. I would just think that I wanted to be away from the pain and, poof, I was free! I didn't know how it was possible, but it was the most exhilarating feeling ever.

My organs were shutting down as I struggled with ARDS and intra-abdominal sepsis. As my fevers raged, my body shook uncontrollably. I felt colder than I thought possible, like I had been dropped into an ice bath in Antarctica with air conditioners blasting at me. My teeth chattered so hard I thought they would crack. I begged for a heated blanket, but I never got one. Apparently the fevers would win if I had one.

As I slipped closer and closer to death, I left my body more frequently. One day, I had enough of the pain and the fever chills and the hopeless feeling of not healing, and I popped out of my body again. Instead of staying in the hospital, though, I found myself in front of a tall, multiple-storied building with two round pillars in front of a tall set of wooden double doors. The building was so high I could not see the top.

It appeared to be crafted from light-colored sandstone, reminiscent of ancient buildings in Jerusalem. Above, the sky stretched wide and bright, a flawless blue without a single cloud, while the sun bathed the scene in warm, golden light—like the comforting heat of a summer afternoon. The area around the building was marked by dusty dirt roads where people slowly wandered as if time had loosened its grip. Dressed in simple beige robes and leather slippers tied loosely around their ankles, they moved with calm ease and an air of quiet reverence, these figures from centuries past. No vehicles disturbed the stillness, and no other buildings broke the horizon, leaving the place suspended in a sacred, timeless silence. It was like stepping into history—where the past and the presence of something divine hung in the air.

As I scanned the area, the building caught my attention again. It exuded a sense of love and peace. I somehow knew that while only the sinless could enter, everyone wanted to be admitted. I felt a magnetic pull toward this building and, without walking through the door, found myself inside. Here I saw people walking and talking quietly. There were a few chairs, and shelves on the walls to my right housed books for people to study. I instinctively knew this building repre-sented knowledge and healing.

Suddenly, my soul found itself in a tall, circular room surrounded by rich, dark, wooden bookcases that stretched upward, like a sacred tower of knowledge. Thousands of leather-bound books in deep reds, worn browns, earthy greens, and faded blues lined the shelves, each one ancient, as if time itself were woven into the very pages.

A warm light filtered down from somewhere above—though I

couldn't see the source—and bathed everything in a gentle, ethereal glow.

This wasn't merely a library—it was a sacred, spiritual archive full of timeless wisdom, a magical sanctuary filled with all the knowledge that ever was and ever would be. Deep, eternal truths whispered from every spine and page. My heart soared at the sight of it all. I have always loved to read, and this room was nothing short of a reader's paradise.

Against the far wall sat a heavy table covered in scrolls that were carefully rolled up and tied with delicate string.

Curious, I moved closer.

Another soul stood next to me. In this realm, or world, souls could understand things about each other without needing to communicate verbally. This soul never said anything, but I could feel his energy, and it felt like he was possibly hundreds or thousands of years old.

He gently picked up a scroll and unfurled the paper. The parchment revealed rows of symbols and ancient writings. I couldn't read the symbols in the way I read earthly words, yet I understood it all, the meaning bypassing my mind and going straight to my spirit. I could have stood here for moments or for eternity, immersed in the divine, never feeling rushed. Time simply didn't exist in this place.

Whatever memories I had as I read the books and scrolls were taken from me when I left this room. I have tried throughout the years to remember the words, but it's like trying to hold water in my hands.

All I know is what I've written here.

Still, somewhere deep within me, I carry the imprint of that knowledge. Even without the details, the feeling remains.

I returned to the main entrance of the building just inside the large front doors. As I stood with my back to them, I noticed off to the right an area with a tall, light-colored, wooden podium and a smaller desk attached to the side that could hold a few small books. There were no seats nearby like you would normally see if someone were giving a speech, so it seemed weird to see this freestanding structure all alone in the middle of the large room. I felt drawn toward this podium, and as I moved toward it, I was delighted to find that I was gliding about an inch above the floor. I remember thinking, *I wish I could move like this all the time!*

As I got closer, the podium lifted off the floor a few inches and slid to the left, revealing a set of stairs to a concealed lower level. No one nearby seemed to acknowledge this was happening as they were involved in other pursuits. I glided toward the stairs, and as I floated down them, the podium closed. I instinctively knew that not everyone was able to enter this area; only certain people were allowed to know it existed.

On the lower level, I entered a vast room filled with pools of shimmering water—an oasis of calm and purity free of anger, hate, and earthly worries. I somehow knew that only the pure of heart could enter this sacred place. To my right stretched a long, rectangular swimming pool, its waters still and deep against a towering wall. To the left, a short waterfall gently cascaded into shallow ponds, their surfaces rippling softly in the tranquil air.

The walls and floors were crafted from sandstone, weathered and timeless, as if shaped thousands of years ago. The space was simple, beautiful, and sacred. The ceiling was high, maybe multiple stories high, and square windows ran along the entire wall a few feet down from this ceiling to let in light. The windows were about two feet by two feet, with about four inches of space between each window. The wall underneath the windows was made of stone. I couldn't see any electricity or plumbing in this large room.

As I took in the scenery, I heard a beautiful sound that calmed my soul in a way nothing ever had. The best I can describe it is water lapping gently against the shores of a still lake. The water called to me, welcomed me. Without hesitation, I went and sat in the nearest pool. The same soul from the great library had accompanied me to this room. He sat nearby, just outside of the water. We had a conversation without needing to use words. It was what I can only describe as a knowledge transfer from soul to soul, where we spoke telepathically. It was like watching a movie that had all the answers to my questions before I asked them. He showed me that this was a pool of healing, living water and that all the water here carried the same sacred, healing power.

A deep and boundless peace washed over me, leaving no room for worry or anxiety—only the embrace of infinite love. In that moment, I was content, safe, and entirely whole. I did not feel any of the pain that had been my constant companion for so long.

As I sat in the large pool, listening to the water lap against the sides, I was mesmerized by the fact that I'd been given the chance to come here to heal. Able to see everything around me in a 360-degree view, I saw myself from above and behind while simultaneously watching the other people playing in the waterfalls and small pools of water. It felt so natural, as if this was how I always saw the world.

While I was in the water, I did not feel wet. My hair and body were dry, but I could feel the water splashing and moving as I ran my hands through the ripples.

To my left, a mother and her two young children, a boy and a girl, jumped up and down and splashed in a waterfall that sparkled like liquid light. I could feel their immense joy. Their laughter rang out in clear, magical bursts, vibrating with happiness as they leaped and twirled through the falling water.

Beautiful rock formations about five to six feet tall framed the waterfall. The water seemed to rise up from the crystal clear pools, then fall from the top of the rocks. Everyone seemed to feel the same euphoric happiness I felt, a happiness devoid of earthly stresses. I closed my eyes and imagined what it would feel like to always be immersed in this healing energy and never have to return to my body.

Eventually, more spirits were allowed to enter. Suddenly, a river of mud came rushing through the walkway, flowed alongside my pool, then passed through a tunnel toward the back of a cave-type area. As the mud rushed by, my friend explained this was because an impure soul had come in and the water turned to mud to expel the unclean soul and purify the area again so it could continue to heal its visitors. After the mud finished flowing through the area, the water became clean and pure again.

During this entire experience, I was never alone. My friend, or Spirit Guide, or the Ancient One, as I had come to think of him, stayed near me, just out of sight, behind my right shoulder, gently explaining and helping me understand what was happening.

Over the next few weeks, I visited multiple times. When I was at my sickest, with fevers dangerously high, I would slip out of my body and find myself in the healing waters. All I had to do was think about the pool, and I was there—effortlessly, instantly, the pain left behind. My soul was whole, and I was able to find some peace away from the chaos of the hospital.

To this day, whenever I am stressed, being in water calms me immediately. For years, I searched for anything remotely close to what I experienced in those healing waters. I eventually found some online pictures of the Church of Saint Anne in Jerusalem, also called the place of healing and mercy. According to tradition, this site marks the home of Anne and Joachim, the parents of Saint Mary, and is believed to be the location of the grotto where Mary, the mother of Jesus, was born. Nearby lies the Pool of Bethesda, mentioned in the Gospel of John as the place where Jesus miraculously healed a paralytic who had suffered for thirty-eight years (see John 5:1–15). The pools were considered medicinal, and many sought healing here. People sat by the pools and waited for a rippling of the water as an angel brought healing to the pool. Tradition said that the first person to jump into the pool was the only one healed. The paralyzed man sat by the pool for thirty-eight years, waiting to be healed. Due to his paralysis, he was never fast enough to be the first in. One day, Jesus came to the man and asked if he really wanted to be healed. When the man said yes, Jesus healed him.

Saint Anne's Church was completed in 1138 by the Crusaders atop the ruins of an earlier Byzantine basilica, which itself had been built over a Roman pagan shrine dedicated to Asclepius, the god of healing. Mind-blowing, right?

In 2022, I saw an online drawing of what many believe Solomon's Temple looked like; it was the closest rendering I have seen to the building I visited. The temple, as described in the Bible, was a grand structure built on Mount Moriah, intended as a dwelling place for the Ark of the Covenant and a place of worship for the Israelites. The temple served as a place for sacrifices, offerings, and prayers and was a symbol of God's presence among His people. After years of trying to explain it with my limited earthly ability, I could finally show others what the outside of the building that held such significance for me looked like.

Of all my near-death experiences, the pools and streams of living water had the most profound healing effect on me. My soul craves the time I spent there. I wish more than anything that I could spend even a single minute in that realm again.

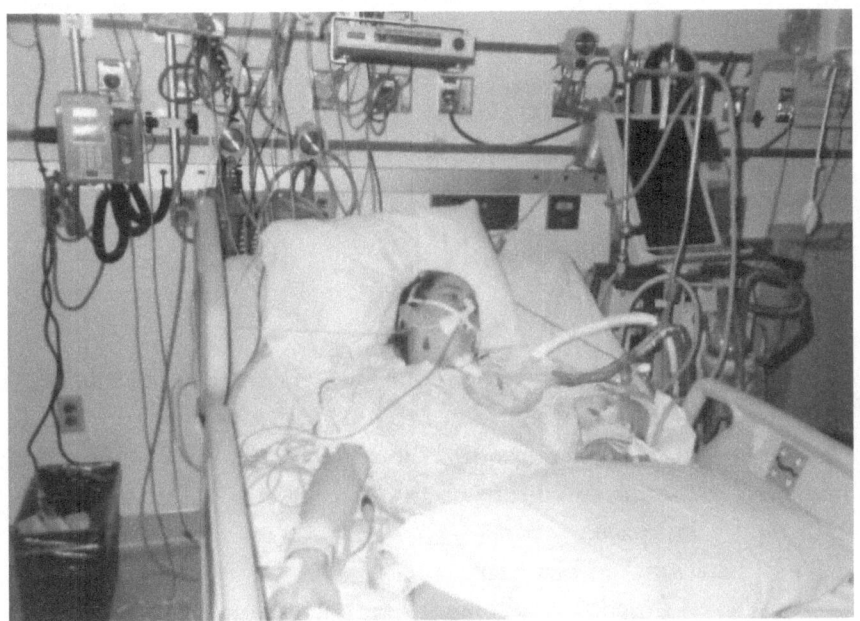

Chapter 8

The Man in a Top Hat: A Fashionable Detour through the Dark Tunnel

It was late at night, and the room was dark, the only visible light coming from my life-support machines. I was lying awake in bed when I felt myself stand up, though standing would have been impossible. Without any means of power, I began traveling upward at an incredibly fast pace.

And there was Top Hat Man.

I was so confused. Everything around me was dark except for this figure.

Yes, I know how that sounds. I was shooting up from the earth in total darkness except for the man next to me, a being surrounded by vibrant light. His dark-brown, kind, soulful eyes looked calmly into mine, his face just a few inches away. He was the only part of this strangeness I was not afraid of. His dark suit with tails and jaunty black top hat made him look like he'd come from the nineteenth century. He wasn't very tall, maybe less than five feet, nine inches, but he reminded me of Abraham Lincoln with his hat, dark facial hair, and white ruffled shirt under the suit coat.

I panicked. I didn't know what was happening or where he had come from. We were traveling so fast that I felt like I was in a speeding car with my head out the window. Yet, even though we hurtled through the darkness, I felt no wind or air. Our clothes were not billowing and our hair was not moving. And the man's top hat stayed in place on his head. It all seemed as if it were perfectly normal for him to come in his 1860s Sunday best to accompany me into the twenty-first century at the speed of light. Maybe he had an explanation, but I didn't think to ask. I was too focused on what was happening.

Time felt suspended. As my panic rose, I popped back into my body so hard it felt like I bounced up off the bed, and then it was over.

This same experience happened a few more times over the next several days, but I never reached whatever was at the end. Each time, I found myself ascending through darkness at what felt like the speed of light. And each time, I became terrified. When I snapped back into my hospital bed, I refused to sleep, afraid that if I closed my eyes, it would happen again.

After three days of this, my nurse noticed I was not sleeping and gave me a shot to sedate me. Being intubated, I couldn't tell them why I wouldn't sleep. These journeys into the unknown began a few days after my January 11 surgery, and the anesthesia from the procedure was fully out of my system, so it was not an effect of the drugs. I was really confused. Looking back, I know this was the tunnel that leads to heaven, the tunnel many who experience an NDE talk about. Even now I do not know who my brown-eyed Abraham was. But he exuded such love and protection that I was never scared of him during these episodes. I have often wondered if he was a distant relative or one of my guides, sent to bring me back home. I should have asked.

Chapter 9

Heaven's Nurses: Angels in the ICU

The next time I left my body, I was transported to a small, rectangular room so tall I couldn't see the ceiling, just white light. This room felt like it was inside the hospital but also not of this realm. Though I couldn't see any light fixtures, the room was bright, the light filling it warm, comforting, and glowing with a calm energy. I noted how different shades of the color white blended together—something I'd never seen on Earth. On the wall to my right was a light-colored wooden door with a square glass window at the top.

Suddenly, I found myself floating about ten feet above the floor. Below, I saw an older man and a plump woman sitting on a long bench. Both had gray hair, and the woman had a bun on top of her head. Both wore light-colored clothing—the woman a light-blue apron with white ruffles and the man a white, button-down shirt paired with light-beige slacks.

These beings emanated such love.

I immediately felt they were guardian angels. When I asked if they were, they explained that they'd been tasked with supporting the critically ill patients in the hospital's shock trauma unit. They spent time in this room, in its Other Side dimension, awaiting their assignments within the earthly hospital.

On their next assignments, they brought me with them. In the trauma unit, we stayed with patients, providing love and comfort. When a patient was not meant to survive, a being I instantly recognized as God would appear—only His face visible through the small glass window at the top of the wooden door leading to the rectangular room.

I knew it was God by the energy radiating from Him. His presence felt powerful and tender and filled with unconditional love and peace. His essence spoke directly to my soul, confirming beyond doubt that this was God, appearing to me just as I needed Him to. I believe He can take on different forms, His appearance reflecting how each person understands or envisions Him, so that when we see Him, we recognize Him with our hearts as much as with our eyes.

And God was truly beautiful. He had a smooth, wrinkle-free face but felt ancient, and He had piercing blue eyes. His silver-and-white, shoulder-length hair and close-shaven beard looked iridescent and glowed like starlight. He exuded an overpowering sense of love and grace, his energy the purest form of that love. I knew He held all the knowledge and love in the universe. I felt safe with Him and was honored that I had been chosen to help these angels as we worked to heal patients and comfort their families.

On one assignment, I stood near an open doorway, looking in on a young man hooked up to a number of life-sustaining machines, including the breathing machine attached to his vent. Just like I had so often been, he was intubated. A few family members, likely his parents and a brother, sat in chairs next to his bed. He was in critical condition, and the two angels with me enveloped him in their love. They also placed their hands on the shoulders of this family to send their love to them. The family never seemed to notice us there, but I know they felt the love we brought.

At one point, after we returned to the rectangular room, I watched as God appeared behind the door, and I knew this young patient was going to pass away. It was then the angels' job to support and comfort the family of the deceased, as well as guide that patient home. When the young man passed, we were there, and our love surrounded his grieving family with comfort and solace.

While we sat in the angels' waiting area, ready to help patients, the angels and I started to talk about my life and what I was going through. I told them I didn't understand how my body was still alive.

"What possible reason is there for me to go through all this if there's no end in sight?"

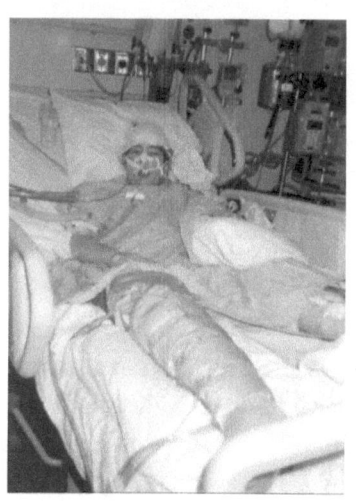

Their answer was puzzling and unexpected. They said that before coming to Earth, I agreed to take on some of the harder trials my youngest brother, Josh, would have had to face in life. This was why I'd had so many setbacks while hospitalized. I was stunned. Josh? At the time, he was still in high school. He didn't seem to have any significant trials. He was a typical teenager with a very easygoing, happy personality and a wide circle of friends. He loved music, especially his favorite rock band, Primus, and went to lots of concerts. I couldn't think of any trials that would be so awful he would need help overcoming them, let alone trials I would need to overcome for him.

Was it possible we agreed to such sacrifices for each other before we even arrived on Earth? How many other invisible acts of kindness played out around us daily?

Many, many years later, my brother's baby boy was born with a serious medical condition we feared might take him from us. As I have watched my brother, a father now, face each situation with courage and tenderness, I have often wondered, *Is this what the angels were talking about?* Maybe, just maybe, some of my brother's life situations could have turned out differently if we had not made the pact we did. My sweet nephew is our little miracle and is thriving at this time, adored and cherished by our entire family.

Chapter 10

Divine Melodies

The music in heaven is unlike anything you'll experience on Earth. On the Other Side, music infuses everything. The water, the trees, the grass—every living thing resonates with a beautiful, harmonious energy. It's as if the entire realm is sustained by these sacred vibrations, each note an extension of divine life and love. Imagine a choir of angels singing melodies so pure, so powerful they don't just echo in your ears, they move through your soul. Each note carries the potential to heal, restore, and awaken something eternal within you. Their music isn't just sound—it's an angelic frequency that uplifts, comforts, and transforms. It's something you cannot hear or feel with your earthly senses. It penetrates your entire being and includes you in its elation.

After returning to my body in the hospital bed one day, I desperately wanted to hear the music that consumed my thoughts. I was intubated at the time and kept trying to communicate with Breezi and my mom that I wanted to hear music. I had a communication chart with a few basic pictures I could point to, plus paper and a pen. My body was weak, and I was hooked up to so many tubes that trying to write a coherent sentence felt frustratingly impossible. My shaking hands could barely hold the pencil. After many tries, I pointed to the radio Matt had brought on Christmas Day, and my mom finally understood.

It was a Sunday morning, and she found a radio station with church music. I was crushed with disappointment. This wasn't anything remotely close to what I had been so lovingly immersed in.

The music I was searching for could be felt with my ears, my heart, my entire soul. It brought me divine, serene peace. Its healing and calming effects kept me moving forward emotionally and spiritually, even if my body wanted to give up. It was so harmonious I craved it with my entire being. The music was similar to the healing waters in the way it healed my broken body and caressed my soul with intense love. It took away my pain, even if for just a few moments.

What I heard on the radio fell far short of what I experienced on the Other Side, making it hard to listen to. The only music remotely close to the heavenly tunes are some types of classical music, especially Bach. When I crave the heavenly voices and instruments, listening to music by Greg Maroney and The Piano Guys, especially "The Cello Song" (Bach's Prelude to Cello Suite No.1 in G Major), can soothe me and bring back that calm, peaceful feeling. Although the music is different from what I remember on the Other Side, I can play these songs, close my eyes, and reconnect with the memories that hold that angelic space in my mind.

Chapter 11

The Last Goodbye

My aunt Alice passed away a few years before my health complications began. Her husband, Harry, lived across the street from my grandparents' house. In life, she was a tiny woman with endless energy. She was no more than five feet tall and had short, curly hair. She wore brightly colored polyester pants and flowery blouses. Despite her energy and cheerfulness, however, she had a fragility about her, probably due to her small stature or the health problems she suffered. Aunt Alice decorated her entire house in Christmas villages each holiday season. For Saint Patrick's Day, she made delicious, green, raisin-filled sugar cookies shaped like four-leaf clovers. Her house was fascinating and fun to explore, and I tagged along with my mom whenever she visited Harry and Alice.

So when Aunt Alice appeared in my hospital room years after her death, I was excited to see her again. At the end of her life, she had been in the hospital ICU. She appeared much healthier on this day than the last time I saw her.

She asked if she could take me back to the house I loved so much, a place that held my childhood memories. I enthusiastically agreed. We just popped into her living room without any effort. It was surreal, like the laws of physics had been bent to allow us this glimpse into a place so dear to me.

The house looked the same as when she was alive, frozen in time. Because she had never updated her house, it was like stepping into the 1970s with its bright-orange, black-speckled countertops; dark wood furniture; knickknacks; and long shag carpet. The old solid-state television encased in its wooden cabinet played quietly from its usual place near the front door in the living room. I found I could see the living room, kitchen, and dining room in a 360-degree view. Since I spent a lot of time here growing up, I felt comforted to be in a familiar place.

As I looked down the hallway just past the dining room and toward the bedrooms, she showed me a sad scene—a place in the hallway where Uncle Harry would fall. No one would be there to help him, and he would ultimately pass away from the complications of this fall. With Aunt Alice gone, Uncle Harry lived alone and was not able to get to a phone to call for help.

I could feel the worry and confusion my uncle was experiencing and knew he felt scared and alone. He couldn't get off the floor by himself. I felt distressed and sad. I didn't want him to die this way! I needed to tell someone to go help him.

After I watched him for a few minutes, I returned to my body. I tried to think of how to find someone to go check on him.

When my family came to visit, I attempted to tell them to go check on Uncle Harry immediately. Since I was still intubated, I tried to write it down on paper, but no one understood. My hands were still too shaky from the pain meds to hold a pencil, so no one could read my scrawl.

I was frustrated that I could not communicate this to anyone. It was like playing charades when no one knew how to play. Eventually, after a few days and many attempts, I was able to relay my concern that he could be dead in the hallway. Someone called Grandpa at home, and he walked across the street to check in on Harry.

He came to the hospital afterward and let me know that Harry was okay and I didn't need to worry. That helped ease my anxiety, but I wondered why Aunt Alice showed me that upsetting scene if my uncle was fine. It didn't make sense.

Harry did end up passing away from a fall in that hallway, but fifteen years later. It was still tragic, but I remember getting the call and feeling validated. It's just that Earth life is bound by time, whereas the Other Side doesn't rely on clocks and calendars like we do.

Chapter 12

Survived Intubation: Still Can't Parallel Park

On the nineteenth of January, my doctors decided to remove my ventilator to see if I could breathe on my own.

My lungs were still damaged, but a ventilator is not something you want to be on long-term. They hoped I would be able to breathe with only the help of an oxygen cannula and that my lungs would grow stronger as I healed. Boy, did I hope so. I hated every minute of intubation. The tubes attached to the ventilator pulled on my face. The one inside my mouth felt suffocating and made it hard to move my head from side to side. Because I couldn't swallow my saliva, a nurse had to suction it to keep me from drowning, which was gross and disgusting. And the tape holding the tubes in place tore my skin. Everything about it was annoying and painful. I felt like I was in a tiny prison, confined to the bed with my face in the even tinier prison of this torturous contraption. The Girl in the Plastic Mask.

I was awake for the removal. And wow—is that even a thing? Watching as they pull this monster out of your throat, inch after inch, longer than you thought possible. And just when you think it's over, they tell you to cough—hard.

They didn't need to tell me twice. It tripped my gag reflex so my cough was genuine and heart (throat) felt! I was so happy it was gone and I could actually talk again.

I didn't realize my vocal cords had been damaged and that I would have to learn how to talk again.

As the nurses cleaned the medical supplies after removing my ventilator, the plain wall opposite my hospital bed transformed. I now saw a beautiful waterfall with gorgeous, lush green plants surrounding it under a sky made of the most vibrant blue. Light shone brilliantly through the blue with a warmth that was a stark contrast to the coldness of my room.

This beautiful scene, like an endless jungle, filled the entire wall from floor to ceiling. Big leafy palm trees and a large waterfall vibrated with living energy, and I could feel within my soul the beautiful music swaying the plants.

This was more like it.

I left my body once again, and as I ventured farther into the jungle. I came upon an open field of grass with a beautiful dwelling in the distance. There was a big wooden barn and water wheel and a cottage near them. They all looked right out of the 1700s. The outside of the cottage was made of large, flat, round rocks, and it had a thatched roof. As water from a small stream poured over the wheel, it collected in wooden buckets that rotated downward and emptied into the pond below. The water bubbling in the pond grew white and foamy toward the edges, reminding me of cream soda bubbling when poured into a cup.

Tall cattails grew around the pond. Like all living things on the Other Side, they seemed to communicate with me, sending me their love.

Without thinking or moving, I found myself sitting on the grass next to the water wheel. I felt a slight breeze, and the soft grass tickled my legs. I was in a place where time didn't exist and I was meant to enjoy this gift of nature.

As fast as I had popped out of my body to sit by the water, I was back in my bed, where everyone was once again unaware that I had left my body.

I was in awe of what I had just experienced but unable to express how beautiful it was. I wanted Mom to experience this amazing reality with me, especially since she and the nurses in my room didn't seem to see what I saw.

As I readjusted to being back in bed, my mom brought me a pink, squishy sponge on a stick to dip into a cup of water to wet my lips for the first time since the removal of my ventilator.

"Now, this is just to wet your lips," said the nurse. "The doctor is worried that if you swallow, you'll aspirate it into your lungs. We have to train you gradually to get back to drinking and eating. It will come in time, but don't gulp anything now!"

My oxygen and ventilator had dried my mouth so much that the water on my lips was like life itself. When Mom held the sponge up to my mouth, I couldn't help it; I sucked the sponge and swallowed. It was the most delicious thing I had ever tasted!

Mom sat down next to me, and I tried to make my voice work, to tell her to look at the beautiful waterfall and to take a sip of this amazing water!

It was cold and wet and flowed over my tongue and down my throat. Nothing could be as delicious as this paper cup of sponge water. I'm not sure Mom could believe me, but it was!

There was no way I was going to let that water cup out of my sight. When no one was looking, I took it off the tray near my lap, dipped the pink sponge into the cup until little pebble ice chips stuck to it, and then sucked on them.

This was one of the first moments of happiness in my hospital room (while in my body!) in weeks. I also felt a little sneaky, and I recognized the return of my stubborn self, which had been missing. It felt good to regain some of the power that had been lost since my hospitalization.

The scene on the wall lasted for less than an hour. No one else could see it, which was a little sad, but it was bright and lovely for me, my room changing from a scary hospital environment to a grounding, healing place in nature.

Chapter 13

Guess Who's Back (Again)

W henever my doctor took me in for emergency surgeries, he told my family he didn't know what he was going to do but would figure it out once he got in there.

On January 26, the doctors discovered five abscesses (pockets of infection) in my stomach. I once again found myself in the cold, sterile operating room for emergency surgery number four, with my doctor slicing open the same incision site to drain the infections.

My skin was so damaged that the surrounding area fell apart as the surgeon made the cut. My internal stitches had started to detach as well. The medical report stated, "We were very worried about the ability of this girl to heal her wound at this point and decided to place retention sutures." Retention sutures are heavy-duty sutures sewn through multiple layers of tissue, including skin, fascia, and muscle. They are tied over a device to distribute the tension and prevent skin damage and are usually removed seven to fourteen days later, unlike sutures, which dissolve on their own. I have many small scars where these were used to *sew* my stomach shut. After the CT scans showed all the infection had been removed and my abdomen had been irrigated and packed internally, I was extubated and transported to recovery.

I received a total of nine blood transfusions due to excessive bleeding during my many surgeries. I was kept in the medical/surgery ICU from January 26 to January 29, where I was in and out of sleep most of the time.

The complications didn't end there.

On January 28, I developed thrombophlebitis—a blood clot—in the PICC line in my right arm. My arm started swelling and hurting, and I called for the nurses. Using ultrasound, they found the clot and decided to remove the PICC line, instead placing a central line into a vein near one side of my collarbone. You'll probably never guess, but that line failed too. I developed a blood infection, and the central line had to be moved to the other side of my collarbone.

My nurses were running out of places to draw blood, which they needed to do multiple times daily to monitor my infections. My nurse mentioned they might need to draw blood from the veins in my legs. I panicked each time the phlebotomists showed up with their vials and needles, and I'd tearfully beg them not to poke me. I was so relieved we never got to the point of leg blood draws and the new central line stayed free of infection.

My surgeon left an eight-inch-long, one-inch-wide incision on my abdomen open throughout my entire hospitalization—and even long after I was discharged. It made it easier when I had to return for emergency surgeries. The nurses packed the incision in gauze that was changed daily to keep it from causing further infections.

My stomach looked hideous. Matt nicknamed it "the baked potato," which I thought was horrible but also, unfortunately, accurate. I didn't eat baked potatoes for a long time after that.

I was on total parenteral nutrition—a feeding tube—my entire hospital stay. And I developed some serious health issues during this time, including diabetes. I had an albumin level between 1.3 and 1.6 grams. A normal adult's is usually between 3.5 and 5.5 grams. Low levels can be a sign of malnutrition and kidney or liver disease, which brings us to the day I met Dr. Vaidya.

~

The fluorescent lights hum softly overhead. Machines beep rhythmically. A dark-haired man in blue scrubs walks into my room. He has a tired face and clutches a clipboard to him like a lifeline.

I lay in bed watching Maury Povich on television. It's getting to the good part. We are going to find out if Tyrell is indeed the father. My hair is a little more wild than usual, my eyes full of mischief and spunk.

"Heather, I am Doctor Vaidya, a surgeon in this hospital. We have run the numbers again. You have chronically elevated liver function tests with alkaline phosphatase documented in the seven hundred to eight hundred range. You have developed sclerosing cholangitis, a disease of the bile ducts. Bile ducts carry bile from your liver to your small intestine. In primary sclerosing cholangitis, inflammation causes scarring within the bile ducts. This scarring makes the ducts hard and narrow, gradually causing serious liver damage. I don't say this lightly —you may need a liver transplant. Soon."

I raise my eyebrows and squint at him. "A liver transplant? Are you sure it's not just . . . having a bad day?"

"Livers don't have bad days. They either work or they don't. Yours is . . . possibly taking an early retirement."

"I know the labs tell one story. But I've been told another story— and I trust the source. The Ancient One said God is going to heal me."

"The Ancient One?"

"Yeah, ya know, my Spirit Guide."

"Heather, I appreciate your faith, but—"

I interrupt him, grinning.

"No, it's more than faith. It's a deep knowing—a certainty that I will be healed and won't need a liver transplant, no matter what the doctors say."

As Dr. Vaidya pinches the bridge of his nose and paces back and forth, looking like he's trying to hold off a migraine.

"You understand this isn't a suggestion. It is life or death."

"Then good news, Doc! I've already been to death. Several times, actually. It's pretty cool!"

He's staring at me. "You do realize this sounds crazy, right?"

"Yup, and I am still the sanest person in this room. God works in mysterious ways, Dr. Vaidya."

Dr. Vaidya mutters something under his breath and scribbles some notes on his clipboard.

"I am going to let you get some sleep. We can discuss this with your family tonight."

As Dr. Vaidya walks out of the room, shaking his head, I wave after him with my yellow-skinned hand. "Wait! Tell the transplant team not to warm up the scalpel just yet. Thank you for stopping by!"

A majority of people with primary sclerosing cholangitis also have an inflammatory bowel disease, such as Crohn's or ulcerative colitis. In most people with primary sclerosing cholangitis, the disease progresses slowly. It can eventually lead to liver failure, repeated infections, and tumors of the bile ducts or liver. A liver transplant is the only known cure for advanced primary sclerosing cholangitis, but the disease recurs in the transplanted liver in a small number of patients.

Ultimately, I did not need a transplant. My liver did indeed heal, just as I promised Dr. Vaidya. And I haven't had any liver complications since. Another divine miracle.

I had gained more than sixty pounds in fluid weight in a very short time. The medication given to reduce the fluid came with side effects and had to be stopped.

The nurses weighed me daily as I lay in bed, unable to move easily because of the many tubes connected to my body. Happily, the bed had a scale that weighed just me and not any of the heavy blankets or medical contraptions on it. That was pretty cool. I liked watching the daily weigh-ins.

I never looked in the mirror because it was like looking at a stranger—a weird, ugly stranger. My feet and hands were so swollen and translucent I thought I would pop. I wasn't able to shower because of the large open wound on my stomach, so the nurses did their best to clean me with a daily sponge bath and dry-shampooed my long hair. My mom braided my hair to keep it out of the way of the tubes taped all over my face. When my long, once-beautiful hair started falling out in large patches and my mom noticed some new gray hairs, I lost even more of my will to live.

Because I wasn't able to move often enough, I continued to develop bedsores on my back. Bedsores are exactly what they sound like, and they are horrible. They cracked and bled, and then the blood dried and glued my back to the sheets. When I moved, the sores opened up and bled. The blood dried into glue again. It was a vicious cycle.

My tailbone, yes, the one that broke just as everything started to spiral, hurt Every. Single. Moment. of Every. Single. Day. The pain was relentless and ever present, a sharp reminder that I was no longer the same person. One day, a nurse showed up with a Polaroid camera to take a picture of the area around my tailbone to track and document things. I already didn't feel human. In a moment of intense humiliation, I watched as she fanned the Polaroid picture of my broken butt, waiting for it to dry. I was a medical experiment no one expected to live. And maybe they were right. The constant setbacks were killing me —killing my will to live.

Chapter 14

Pop-Up Docs and Near-Death Shocks

As the snow fell outside my hospital window, I suddenly found my soul floating above a vast field bathed in summer's golden warmth. The field stretched endlessly, lush and full of life, long blades of grass in various shades of green dancing and swaying in the soft breeze. Tall oak trees towered, reaching for vivid blue skies. A few small fluffy white clouds drifted lazily about.

In the distance, I noticed a cluster of white tents with long white tables inside them in the middle of the field. I floated down toward the tents like an invisible force and entered without hesitation. Inside, a group of doctors in crisp white lab coats worked quietly together.

The environment was full of tension and stress. They worked rapidly and quietly in sync, writing notes, reading medical books, and using microscopes to look at the contents of various petri dishes. The doctors were engrossed in their work and didn't notice me—or the figure standing just behind my right shoulder. Though I couldn't see him, I felt his familiar presence. It was my Spirit Guide, the Ancient One, who had been with me all along.

I didn't recognize any of the doctors in the tent. I felt like I had been brought here to help me understand what my actual doctors were thinking and feeling as they tried to heal me. I got the impression that my doctors were under a fast-approaching deadline and needed answers.

As I watched them, my Spirit Guide and I began to engage in a silent, spiritual dialogue. He said, "They don't know how to heal you. It is only through faith and the prayers of others that you will survive."

Up to this point, I had relied on the doctors to "fix me," and now, hearing that there was a plan at work to save me helped take away some of the fear I felt as I moved toward death. It also made my laughter at the liver doctor make more sense. Some part of me knew that healing would come in ways my medical team could not envision.

Maybe these doctors were here to show me that the Other Side was assisting my earthly doctors from beyond? I had started to doubt I could come back from my medical complications without any serious health concerns. My mom started praying I would die and be released from my hellish nightmare. She said it was too painful to watch her child suffer, helpless to save me, and so she asked for my release. No parent should ever have to watch their child die slowly, unable to help them. It was a cruel paradox: her love for me, her agony over watching me suffer, and my inability to forever leave my earthly body behind.

Unknown to me, during this time, my parents' church congregation had gathered to fast for twenty-four hours and then went to their chapel the next night to pray for me.

Throughout my illness, various neighbors and friends would visit us at the hospital and ask my parents how they could help. But everyone felt so helpless. My parents could only tell them to pray that I would either be healed or allowed to pass quickly and peacefully.

I truly feel that God hears our prayers, sent like balls of light, full of love, to our Creator. He doesn't always answer them the way we wish, but each and every prayer is heard.

I know God heard the many heartfelt prayers offered on my behalf throughout my hospitalization. I am here today because of those prayers.

Chapter 15

Over My Dead Body

I tried not to pop out of my body when any of my nurses or family were present because I didn't want to scare them. But sometimes it happened anyway. One day, when my mom and nurse were getting me ready for my daily walk, the burning in my stomach and the fevers became too much, and I left again. I found my soul in a hallway, one that seemed to stretch on for eternity, a brilliant light at the other end. The light was almost blinding, but it did not hurt my eyes. Tall, arched windows lined both sides, spaced every few feet. Beneath each window, a low ledge offered just enough room for a small child to sit on.

In this hallway, to my right, I could see my hospital room with my body sitting up and my legs dangling over the side of the bed. I faced my nurse, Brian, who stood a few inches from my face and held me upright by my shoulders. My mom was also in the room, partially behind him.

Brian was saying, "Come back, Heather. Come back!" He waved one hand in front of my face while holding my shoulder with the other, snapped his fingers, asked how many fingers he held up, and called my name again and again.

I was sitting upright, but my body wasn't reacting—my face was blank, my eyes unblinking, and I sat completely still, as if frozen in time. My chest was not rising and falling. I was staring at my empty earthly body with no desire to go back to that heavy, painful shell.

Brian pleaded with me to come back. Mom looked so helpless, so fragile, the intensity of my health problems visible in her face, in the stoop of her shoulders. She spent every minute of every day trying to take care of me while still working full-time at her job. Her three teenage boys at home also relied on her. She was losing weight because she was too upset to eat and didn't have time to prepare meals when she did have an appetite. All her spare time was spent with me, and taking care of herself was not a priority. I didn't want to watch my mom suffer if she lost me at that moment. I watched the scene unfold for a few minutes while I battled internally about what I should do. I felt so peaceful away from that body but worried about my mother and Brian, who really didn't want me to die under his care. I eventually decided to return to my body, knowing that once the room was quiet, I would pop back out of my body again to return to my pain-free haven.

When my soul returned to my body, I felt disoriented and upset that I was back and in pain again. Brian looked me in the eye and asked, "We lost you there for a minute! Do you know where you are? What year is it?" and all the other coherence questions I was sick of having to answer.

I wanted to scream, "Yeah, you did lose me! It was *great*! Why did you make me come back?"

I hated being imprisoned in a body so broken and pain-ridden. I kept hoping that, at some point, I would leave my body for good and live fully in the bliss and happiness of the Other Side. I didn't want my family to be sad if I left, but I also knew that if I was given a choice to stay or go, I would join my grandparents and aunt on the other side, not giving any thought to the feelings of those I left behind.

I wanted to be forever immersed in the love I felt there.

Years later, I mentioned this day to my mom. She said that when Brian sat me up, I looked empty and lifeless, like I wasn't there. As Brian pleaded with me to come back, she felt helpless seeing how sick I was and didn't know how I had survived up to that point.

She had hoped I would be released from my pain and pass on.

I asked if she discussed with any of the nurses what they saw when I was not present in my body. Mom said they only talked about the medical side of my treatment and wouldn't discuss anything outside of that.

Chapter 16

The Window Between Worlds: A Glimpse of the Divine

While in my hospital bed one day, I saw a figure I immediately recognized as Jesus. He stood just outside my hospital window, visible from His chest up, looking into my room. Six floors up. I pointed to the window and said, "Look, I see Jesus at the window."

I did not have a problem with Him being outside my window. When I wasn't in my body, I could float too. If I was able to float, Jesus definitely could. He looked very different from God. He had darker hair and eyes, a thinner face, and His own energy. His eyes seemed to hold all the love and pain in this world. I felt a deep sense of familiarity, like we were family, together since long before this lifetime. I was in awe that He cared enough to check in on me, and I felt such immense love radiating from Him. I wanted to stay with Him forever. I wished He would gather me in His arms and tell me He was here to take me home, ending my pain and suffering.

Unfortunately, that did not happen. He was gone as fast as He appeared.

Although His time with me was brief, it gave me hope that I would either die or He had come to heal me. I hoped to receive an answer soon.

When my mom looked at the window, she couldn't see Him. She saw only the snowy landscape and the reflection of her daughter, who was slipping away. My family was under an immense amount of stress. I can only imagine how unsettling it was hearing me talk about dead relatives and Jesus.

Seeing these spirits, however, comforted me and helped me feel less alone. They felt like "home" to me. Seeing souls from the Other Side helped my mind calm down and not focus on the pain because they brought a beautiful healing energy that made me forget my worries.

I hovered between two worlds, my family clinging to the one where I still breathed and lived.

Chapter 17

Caring Hearts, Healing Hands

During the day, my room was alive with activity and noise, and I never felt alone.

Nights were entirely different. The hospital felt dark and scary even though there were always lights in the hallways and at the nurses' station.

It seemed like every time I drifted off to sleep, I heard a loudspeaker announce a code blue. My machines beeped so loudly that I found it hard to settle down, and I cried from the fear and pain.

I had a few wonderful nurses who sat with me when they had extra time during their shifts. We never talked about the elephant in the room—my medical issues with their very real possible side effect, death. Instead, they caught me up on current events or asked me about my life before hospitalization. We talked about family holiday traditions, favorite books and foods, and the best places to vacation.

One nurse knew how much I wanted to have an actual shower instead of a sponge bath. I had been in the hospital for over a month at this point without one actual shower. She received permission from my surgeon for a one-time shower with a detachable spray-hose nozzle.

I had won the lottery. I had been confined to my bed besides the few minutes each day when my doctor required me to walk the length of the hallway to prevent blood clots.

I was normally too sick to care, but when I was conscious enough to notice, I really missed the feeling of hot, cleansing water. So I couldn't believe my luck and the thoughtfulness of this nurse. She helped me wrap my entire stomach with Saran Wrap to keep water from getting inside my wound. Then I had to be wheeled to a special shower room with a tiled, flat-entry shower large enough to fit my two IV poles and medication bags that were coming along for the ride.

After she positioned me on a hospital shower chair, she took a seat across from me and held my arm to keep me upright. With her other hand, she sprinkled the warm water over my legs, arms, and hair, carefully avoiding the parts of my body that could not get wet.

The water felt heavenly on my rough skin, healing and cleansing it like the waters on the Other Side. Tears streamed down my face, mingling with the shower water. For something previously so simple and part of my everyday routine, which had been absent for too long, it felt like sensory overload. The nurse didn't rush me, either. She let me bask in this experience for as long as I was able to sit up. As she showered me, she told me about her day and what was going on outside the hospital. I wanted to hear it all. I loved intelligent conversations that were not all about how imperiled my life was. They were just the best. She understood that. She treated me like I was a real person worth the conversation, not just a half-dead patient.

For whatever reason, this shower gave me hope that maybe I could eventually be well enough to do a few tasks on my own. It helped me feel human again. Being able to talk about anything besides medical jargon—even something as simple as the latest TV show or the weather—was a relief. That small moment of compassion was more healing than any medication.

I will always be grateful beyond words for this nurse, for the care she showed me that day and every day she was involved in my care. Regretfully, I cannot recall her name, which really bothers me. I can see her smiling face so clearly, surrounded by shoulder-length, dark-brown hair, her voice so calming. She helped me feel safe in a very chaotic situation. I nicknamed her my angelic nurse, a title she more than earned.

Chapter 18

Heaven's "Not Yet": A Return I Didn't Choose

L eaving my body yet again, I found myself in a place that felt sacred—an area with hundreds, possibly thousands, of spirits lining an entrance, facing each other across a soft cloud-like path that stretched far beyond them.

The only way I can think to describe this area is to have you imagine you are outside on a foggy day, but warm sunlight filters through the mist, and everything is alive and full of warmth and love.

The clouds, in golden tones of yellow mixed with iridescent layers of white, blanketed the ground, and I thought to myself how interesting it was that we were all able to stand on them and not fall through. They felt so solid.

For as many different souls as were in this area, it was strangely quiet, like a snow globe after you shake it and everything settles down, leaving a beautiful, silent scene. Perfect.

The energy here was strong, vibrating in waves of love. The beings were so brilliantly lit I could not distinguish any facial features, only the vibrant light that surrounded them. They were all different heights, barefoot, and dressed in thin white-beige robes that also glowed with this light. They stood so close their bodies merged into one endless chain stretching beyond sight.

Then, in an instant, I knew. I *knew* them. All of them. They were relatives and friends from different generations who had previously passed and were there to welcome me home. They knew me too. I felt their love and recognition. It felt like an honor guard of souls, welcoming, loving, and deeply familiar.

I knew I was at the entrance to heaven not because anyone told me but because it felt familiar, like returning home after a long time away. The peace there was more profound than anything I ever experienced on Earth. I had expected a golden gate at the entrance to heaven, but there wasn't one, just a seamless, open space that seemed to welcome me from beyond.

And somehow, I understood the *rules*. I knew if I crossed that invisible threshold, there was no coming back. I wouldn't return to my family or my earthly problems. I would be forever free.

My Spirit Guide, my constant companion, stood in his usual place.

I thought, *I'm going to tell the Ancient One I am going to visit my grandma and her garden and then come back, even though I'm not ever coming back.*

Yes, I know. I was planning something in my head when "inside my head" was a wide-open book on the Other Side.

Still, I plotted to sneak into heaven without anyone noticing. I knew it was of the utmost importance that I pass through that entrance as fast as possible to be home-free and never return to my broken body.

I was in the fiercest competition of my life and had to win at all costs, with stakes higher than anything I ever faced. There was no room for surrender, no hesitating. The calm and warmth of heaven beckoned.

As I thought this, the Ancient One spoke. "You have to go back. It is not your time yet."

I felt devastated. I may have thought of a swear word. Maybe two.

I did *not* want to go back to Earth, and I would have given anything to be able to stay there, forever floating in a vast sea of energetic love.

But poof! I was back in my body. I felt like I had blown my last chance to exit this life and return home. I lay there, stunned and heavy with disappointment. I had been so close. Being pulled back felt like a cruel trick.

The only time I truly felt "alive" was when I was out of my body, and each time I visited the Other Side, I became less attached to my body and my life here. I felt less and less tethered to the fragile shell that imprisoned my soul.

Looking back, I find it funny that I thought I could fool my guide, because he *knew* me. He knew my thoughts as soon as I formed them in my mind. I'm sure he got a good laugh out of me trying to pull a fast one on him.

Chapter 19

A Divine Glimpse into My Future

As my days in the hospital wore on, two children and a man began appearing in my room, standing at the foot of my bed, not having come through the door. They never said anything. Sometimes the boy came alone, and sometimes he brought the girl and an older man dressed in a light-gray suit.

The first time they visited while my mom was there, I said rather casually to her, "There are the kids again."

My mom looked startled. "What kids?"

I didn't understand why she could not see the two children. They were so obviously at the foot of my bed, plain as day.

"The two kids. Boy and a girl. They come and stand at the foot of my bed. Sometimes they bring an older man with them."

Mom looked at the place where I could see them but she couldn't. "Do you think the man is your grandfather?"

"I don't know, Mom. I can't remember him so well. The kids have hazel eyes and blond hair. The boy's hair is curly, and the girl's is straight. They don't talk or anything. They just watch me."

She nodded slowly, her face etched in confusion, but said nothing more that day.

Over time, their presence felt less like a mystery and more like a comfort. I never felt scared. In fact, they brought a stillness with them, like they held space for me between two worlds, as if they waited for me, guarding the veil.

Matt and I joked about these encounters, wondering who these two children were and why they came. Both Mom and Matt suggested that the children were our future kids. But, of course, they couldn't be. My hair is brunette, and Matt is Portuguese. How could we be the parents of two blond, hazel-eyed children?

How could I think about being a mother when I couldn't even take care of myself? And pregnancy was absolutely impossible.

And, just like that, one day, they stopped appearing.

Maybe they finally knew I was going to stay.

Chapter 20

From The Other Side With Love

At one time, after returning to my body, I told my parents that I had been with my grandma who had passed away a year before.

"She told me I would be okay. I just needed to eat." I couldn't tell them any more, though, as I could only remember her telling me to eat and not how I'd heal. I became upset because I'd wanted to go on with her after I was sent back to earth life. I didn't want to answer any more questions that day.

I was still in fairly critical condition at this point, and Matt and my parents must have thought I was crazy to think that eating would cure me.

~

The next time my grandpa came to visit, I lay in my hospital bed, the sun casting rays of light across my blanket through the blinds.

Grandpa pulled a chair up next to my bed and sat down, grabbing my hand.

He looked tired but sharp and steady.

"Grandpa," I said quietly. "I saw Grandma. I was with her when I left my body."

He stared at me for a minute, quietly digesting the information, then swallowed back his tears. "I miss her so much. Tell me about your time with her. Did she say anything about me?"

I thought about my time with her, feeling her love engulf me once again.

"She radiated love, Grandpa. She watches over our family. She's been aware of our lives since her passing. She told me I will be healthy again"

He nodded slowly, his face raw with emotion, his eyes glistening with tears.

"Tell her . . . tell her I love her and have never stopped. I don't want to leave you, but she is my first and last thought each day. I can't wait to see her again. She took part of me with her when she left."

My grandmother's passing had been fast, unexpected, and devastating. She was the glue that held our family together. She remembered every single birthday, cooked homemade meals for every holiday, and made me feel like I was her favorite grandchild. Being back in her comforting embrace on the Other Side, the same arms that held me as a child, was indescribable. I was home in the most eternal way. I felt completely safe, completely known, completely engulfed in the ever-present love of my childhood.

My recovery was much more complex than this, but eating was integral to my healing as I lost so much weight over the next few months. My body wasn't retaining nutrients, and my nutritionist was having my nurses add extra Ensure to my feeding tube to help me gain the weight I kept losing. Daily, the nurses weighed me and then adjusted the medications and tube feeding based on what the readings showed. When I did eat actual food, my stomach became full really fast and hurt all the way up into my rib cage. That made it hard to breathe, so I only ever took a few bites before pushing the food away.

As my time in the hospital wore on, I memorized the hospital lunch and dinner menu rotation. Each day, a card with the menu showed up with my breakfast tray in the morning, and I could choose meals for lunch and dinner. I had been vegetarian since age twelve and found a few meals I really liked, especially the mashed potatoes, rice pilaf, and warm veggie broth.

The worst food the cafeteria ever served was the scrambled eggs molded like a small loaf of bread with syrup poured over them. It was disgusting. I couldn't figure out what kind of maniac would serve that to anyone, let alone someone with limited moments of joy.

They put me on a semisoft diet after my ventilator was removed, and new foods were slowly introduced to see how I reacted.

When Matt visited at night, he grabbed dinner from the cafeteria and sat with me while he ate and watched wrestling or some other loud TV show. He brought food that was not on my approved list, and I practically drooled as he stuffed his face with forbidden nachos. I felt a feral longing for fast food, which I was never a big fan of before that point. Having the same few soft, dull foods every day got really boring.

One day when Matt stepped out to grab a drink, he left his nachos sitting on the wheeled hospital tray propped over my bed. As soon as he walked out, I grabbed a chip with extra cheese sauce on it and took a bite before anyone could catch me. The chip had been sitting in a pool of the hot, melted, gooey cheese sauce and had turned soggy.

It was absolutely the most delicious thing I had eaten in months. I wanted to eat the entire plate, but I didn't know if my stomach could handle more than one chip after such a long stretch of bland food. Plus, having a nurse walk in as I inhaled the chips and drank the cheese sauce was a bad look.

Before Matt returned, I went in for one more glorious chip—this time with an extra scoop of golden cheese. I savored the victory as I crunched it down like a stealthy snack ninja. When he came back, he didn't notice the two missing chips or the smug little grin I wore like a badge of honor.

I was so tired of being told what I could and could not eat, I resolved I would get better so I could get rid of my feeding tube. I vowed, like Scarlett O'Hara, that as God was my witness, I *would* sit down in front of a feed trough of spicy, greasy, deep-fried, bean-smothered cheese burritos and not share a single one! I had to dream of something, and this was a good dream.

Chapter 21

When You Leave Your Body But Still Micromanage Your Family

With each new day I spent in the hospital, I became more homesick. I wanted to go home and never step foot in another hospital again.

It was starting to feel like I would live at the hospital forever.

Every time I thought about it, I became depressed and anxious. Breezi worked nearby and visited often. I could hear her cheerfully saying hello to the nurses outside my room before she entered. She'd bring me silly stories from work along with her calming presence. We'd laugh about old memories and talk about anything but the hospital. For a few precious moments, I didn't feel sick. She'd sit by my bed, crack jokes, update me on mutual friends, or just hold my hand as I drifted in and out of sleep. I looked forward to her visits each day. I don't think she truly knew how much those moments meant to me.

My nurse mentioned one day that patients could receive special permission to bring their animals to the hospital when they were at the end of their life. She asked if Matt would like to bring my two cats. She said it brought comfort to patients to hold their animals one last time before they passed. She made it sound final, but I was intrigued.

Mom was horrified. She told the nurse it was not a good idea to bring dirty animals into a sterile hospital when I was so sick and could possibly get another bacterial infection. I knew that puppies were brought into the hospital to lift patients' spirits, but they were on leashes, and I didn't want to worry about my cats getting loose and running amok. I could picture them arriving, fur puffed, eyes wild, yowling as they scraped their way out of Matt's arms and escaped into the halls of the ICU like tiny little panthers. No, thank you. No one needed that kind of chaos. The cat discussion was shelved faster than you can say "hiss," and no one ever brought it up again.

The nurses were ever in and out of my room, drawing blood, taking vitals, and wheeling me down for MRIs and CT scans. My sleep rhythm was so far off it didn't exist. I took short naps throughout the day and night whenever I could.

One night, as I lay awake staring at the ceiling, I left my body and found myself flying over the city.

As it was the middle of the night, it was dark outside but clear and beautiful. I could see all the stars twinkling in the sky as well as all the lights from the buildings and houses.

The noise of traffic and daily life were gone as most people were home asleep.

I felt an incredible sense of freedom to not only be out of my body again but from the sheer joy of moving so effortlessly through the sky. I had always said if I could have one superpower, it would be to fly. And here I was, soaring. I wasn't sure where I was being taken, but I didn't care. Rooftops passed by in a blur. I felt so light and untethered.

After what felt like five minutes but was probably much longer, I ended up in the front entryway of my house, and all my feelings of being homesick vanished. I noticed I had not needed to use the front door, and that felt pretty magical. We had a classic split-level home, the kind where you can either go up or down the stairs when you enter the front landing area. I was near the top of the ceiling above the entrance. At the top of the stairs, I could see my two cats, Snickers and Twix, curled next to each other, sleeping.

I stayed above them for a few minutes, then thought I should check on Matt. The instant I had that thought, I drifted down the hall and gazed into our bedroom through the open door, watching from a quiet vantage point near the ceiling. Matt lay asleep in bed on his side, facing the window with our comforter covering his body and his favorite blanket, Blue Blanks, near the top of his head.

As I watched him sleep, I felt a voice whisper that a nurse was coming into my room and it was time to return.

I did not fly over the city again but popped back into my body like so many times before.

Being able to go home for a few minutes reduced my anxiety and helped me feel like, one day, I would be able to leave the hospital and go back to who I was before all this happened. It reinforced that I did have a life and a home to return to.

Chapter 22

Family Reunions: Orb Edition (Less Awkward than the Family BBQ)

W hen I was little, my grandma Ardell took me with her whenever she visited her dad, my great-grandpa James. He lived forty-five minutes away, and we spent the drive listening to Big Band music from the 1940s.

I loved Great-Grandpa James's place. It was an older brick home with an arched front door and a kitchen fireplace surrounded by brick. It was so welcoming and always filled with my grandma's sisters and brothers and their kids, who stopped over when we visited. He had a one-acre garden in his backyard with a canal behind the garden that all the grandkids liked to play in. And he made the most delicious soup with tomatoes, zucchini, carrots, potatoes, and many other vegetables from his garden. He served it with hot, fresh, buttered bread we ate at the kitchen table. Great-Grandpa was active in his garden until he passed at age ninety-four, when I was ten years old.

Losing him was hard on my grandma, who missed him terribly after he passed on.

About three weeks into my hospital stay, I found myself in my grandma Ardell and grandpa Howard's backyard on their stone patio, facing the back of the yard.

I spent countless hours of my childhood here, sitting on metal rocking chairs holding my infant cousins, chasing my older cousins as we played tag, and sharing family dinners on this patio.

It was wonderfully comforting to be somewhere so familiar.

As I looked toward the back of the yard above the clothesline, I noticed orbs of light floating across the yard from right to left. They were about seven to eight feet above the ground and varied in size. There were ten to twelve in total, the largest the size of a basketball, others a mini watermelon, and the smallest the size of an apple. Some of the orbs were full of darker blue-and-green light with a silver, glitter-like color that floated around inside of the orb, and they seemed to be spreading love as they passed by. They reminded me of the glittery liquid inside a lava lamp.

In one orb, I saw the familiar face of Grandma Ardell, her expression radiating pure love. Two larger orbs followed, revealing the glowing faces of my great-grandpa James and my aunt Alice. They looked the same as they had near the time of their passing—only healthier and brighter looking, illuminated by the light. Recognition washed over me, especially for my grandma and aunt, who had been regulars in my out-of-body experiences. But this was the first time seeing my great-grandpa. It felt like a warm embrace after ten years apart.

They drifted slowly to the left, gliding beyond the lush garden, past my grandpa's woodshop. I wanted to follow, to stay in their presence a little longer, but my feet stayed rooted to the ground as they gently faded from view.

Although the night sky was dark, the area surrounding the orbs glowed softly, illuminated by dozens of stars. It was completely silent —no barking dogs, no wind, not even a whisper of movement. Time felt suspended, as if it didn't exist at all. I saw no one else, yet I knew I wasn't alone. The Ancient One stood nearby, a quiet presence watching over me with calm, protective strength.

I accepted all this as if it were an everyday occurrence. I felt loved and protected, and I enjoyed being in a place that had such a positive impact on my childhood and held so many of my favorite memories. Once the orbs disappeared, I calmly returned to my body in the hospital.

Chapter 23

Don't Mind Me—Just Coming and Going as I Please

As the days went on and I continued my stay at "Hotel Hospital," my family felt it would be best if a family member or close friend was with me as often as possible so we could get updates from the doctors after rounds and keep an eye on my condition. Matt would sit with me and watch TV as I drifted in and out of sleep.

He later told me I would have my eyes closed as I slept but would suddenly jolt awake. I would look shocked for a minute, like I was trying to figure out where I was as I came back to reality. When he asked me if I was okay, I would give him a blank, disoriented look. He said it was like I had to reintegrate with my body and the hospital room again. It usually took me a few minutes to be fully "back" in the present.

Because I was attached to so many life-support machines in addition to the PICC line in my arm or clavicle, I couldn't move around unless a nurse helped me. I was mostly quiet during this time of my hospitalization due to my ventilator and too tired to listen to conversation for more than a minute. Besides vitals checks, blood draws, and imaging, I was mainly left to heal as I slept, which made it easier for me to leave my body when the pain became unbearable.

My mom visited me every morning before work, during her lunch break, and every night after work. My dad took FMLA (unpaid leave) from his job with the federal government at the local Air Force base and spent the days sitting in the chair next to my bed, reading his leather-bound Louis L'Amour books while I drifted in and out of sleep.

My dad is a quiet person who doesn't show emotion easily, but he showed his love by being there every day and making sure I received the best possible care.

During moments of quiet, I would look over at my dad to make sure he was engrossed in his books. And then I would pop out of my body. I had no control over what happened to me when I was in my body, but once out, I could shed the heaviness and move freely. While on the Other Side, I didn't have the usual worries I did on Earth. I felt like I was home after a vacation to a weird country where the only constant was pain. I craved the peace and the love-filled, care-free environment. I wanted to find a way to stay on the Other Side because when I was there, I could be the me that felt most like my authentic self.

In my body, I couldn't sit up on my own, let alone walk, without two nurses holding me up. I was in complete survival mode and desperately unhappy, just trying to get through each day without so much as moving. I tried to hold still so I wouldn't snag any of the wires or tubes attached to me. Nurses still moved me to other positions throughout the day so I would not get more bedsores. I dreaded it so much that I cried every time it happened. They really did try to be as gentle as possible; it wasn't their fault it hurt. They knew what to do, grabbing the bottom sheet on both sides and using it to move me farther up the bed whenever I slid down. Unable to help them with this simple task, I felt like a teary, sobbing blob of Jell-O as I slid all over the bed. My stomach incision again felt like it was on fire, and it was too hideous to believe it was part of me; it looked like a wounded sea creature.

Once I was transferred out of shock trauma to the heart and lung critical care unit, Dr. Pearce, my lung doctor, ordered me to walk each day, even if just from the bed to the door, to prevent blood clots. There was a dry-erase board on the wall with my nurse's name and other important information. It also listed the times for my daily walk. I hated that board. I'd make myself sick anticipating the next round, dreading the moment I'd once again feel like I was being dragged helplessly around the room like a wounded—yeah. That.

Every day, sometimes twice a day, it took two nurses ten minutes to detach my life-support machines, other medical devices, and medication bags from the bed and wall and attach them to an IV pole or my walker. The nurses set me in a wheelchair while they transferred all this stuff to the chair and poles, then changed my bedding. After that, they stood on either side of me and, holding me under both my scrawny arms, lifted me off the wheelchair. With every nerve on fire, I tried not to call them terrible names. I died from humiliation, pain, and rage as they helped me try to walk with my walker.

Every step I took had me crying in pain and desperation while everyone else in the room cheered me on. Multiple J-tubes draining my infections dangled from my stomach. Heavy and awkward, they swung back and forth, the tape securing them to my body pulling away and ripping layers of my skin off. Hovering around eighty to ninety pounds, I did not have skin to spare.

Dad joined me and the nurses, helping to hold me up as I struggled through the torture. It also took forever because I frequently had to stop and catch my breath.

If my favorite nurse was on shift, he'd stride into my room with the energy of someone who took his coffee intravenously. He'd look at my dad, flash a grin, and loudly announce, "Let's get this revelry started!"

Then came the fanfare.

He'd cup his hands around his mouth and belt out enthusiastic noises that sounded like he was playing a trumpet. It was gloriously ridiculous. My dad, usually solemn and quiet, cracked up every time.

This rambunctiousness woke me every single time, letting me know it was time to walk the halls.

One morning during this nurse's usual performance, my surgeon happened to be in the room, checking on his star patient.

At the sound of the impromptu trumpet blast, his head jerked up, his eyes wide, his mouth agape. Then he smiled and shook his head.

If the nursing gig didn't work out, my nurse had a job waiting in medieval pageantry.

As goofy as he was, that silly little ritual got me up and walking.

~

One of my lowest lows came after my fourth abdominal surgery. No one knew it had happened until it was time to walk the floor, but during the surgery, I had been positioned incorrectly on the table. When it came time for my walk, my foot was dragging, but no one noticed because of my long hospital gown. My body had become so atrophied and it took so much effort to put one foot in front of the other that as I tried to lift my left leg forward, that foot lagged behind me like something dead. But it did not feel dead; it felt like the muscle attaching the top of my foot to my leg had snapped. It was no longer lifting my foot as I walked, and it was agonizing. As we moved through the door to leave my room, my nurses moved forward to give me space to get through, but my foot was all wrong, so I fell inside my walker and landed on the ground, getting tangled in some of my tubes in the process. That tube tangle prevented me from going all the way down. Instead, I just dangled there, half hanging on to my walker, half on the ground. Everyone rushed to pick me up, but I felt so beaten and pathetic I wanted to get back to my bed to rest.

Learning how to walk again began that day. To regain the use of my left foot and leg, I had to go to physical therapy four times a day. PT happened in a room with torture—I mean exercise—equipment, where I sat on a pedal machine with my feet strapped down, and tried with all my might to pedal one time around the wheel.

Every single minute of that time sucked. It sucked so bad. Wore me all the way out. Man, I hated physical therapy. I can't even remember how many times my physical therapist had to help me push my legs to get the bike to spin. My tailbone was still damaged, painful, and swollen. It hurt so bad when I sat down on that hard seat. I was in hell and always relieved when my therapy session ended and they let me go back to my room to sleep.

I will happily say that the nurses who attended to me during this time were amazingly gentle and patient as I worked to regain my strength. I owe them a lot of my survival.

Because of the incorrect positioning during that last surgery, I developed what they called "foot drop." I could have told them that, but they officially determined it with more tests. It's self-explanatory for the most part. My foot dropped. The wonky position the foot was in during surgery caused some pretty severe nerve damage. It took years to feel like my left leg and foot were equal to my right instead of being hit with a million flaming little needles whenever anything touched it.

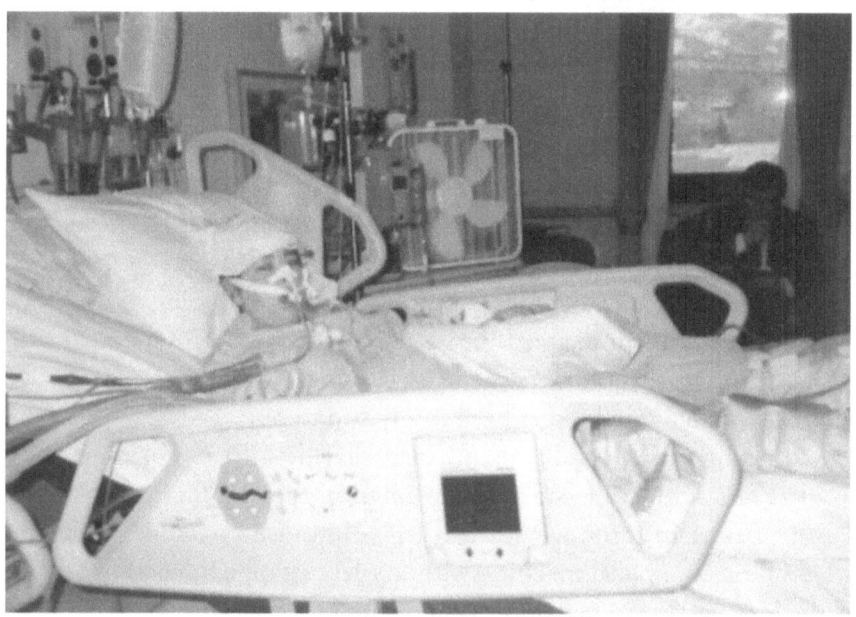

My dad hiding in the background, reading his book and eating lunch.

But then, miracle of miracles, after years of hardly daring to dream of a normal foot, it healed enough that I could finally entertain the thought of a pedicure. It had been years.

The timing couldn't have been more perfect. I had just bought the perfect pair of sandals—white, strappy, and begging for brightly colored toes. On a sunny afternoon, I decided it was time to bravely face my fears. I confidently walked into the salon, half expecting to bolt once the nail tech touched my foot.

"Treat yo'self, girl." I half whispered to myself with a little smirk as I looked for the perfect color of polish on the shelves.

The foot soak in warm sudsy water felt like a five-star spa experience. When the nail tech scrubbed my foot, I giggled—it tickled! It didn't shoot sharp pricks of pain up my leg. I wanted to throw confetti.

And the color—it was sparkly, unapologetically pink, like cotton candy got promoted. It was ridiculous and fabulous and exactly what I needed.

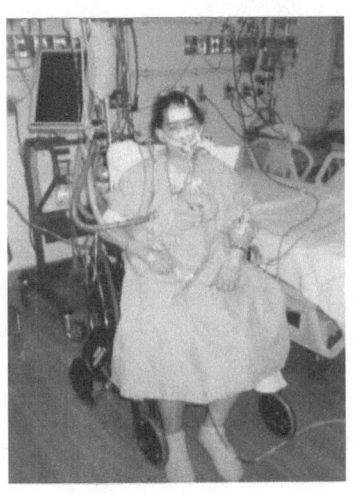

When she finished, I couldn't stop staring at my toes. This wasn't just a pedicure; it was a celebration. A comeback tour. A victory. I felt fabulous and full of life again!

In my excitement, I tipped way more than 20 percent without a thought.

No one in the salon knew what a big deal that day was for me.

Getting ready to walk the halls with all my medical equipment.

I strutted out of the salon like I was on my own personal runway, the midday sun sparkling almost as much as my pink toes.

Victory.

Chapter 24

I'm Not Dead, Just Resting

Matt's grandmother, Grandma Dar, frequently visited the hospital. We were very close, and she was distraught that I was so sick. She would sit next to my bed and try to rub any part of my arm not connected to IVs and other medical devices. She sometimes stayed for hours, telling me she needed me to fight and not die.

I had no desire to live and loved the Other Side. It was truly my home, but she was so sweet I couldn't tell her.

One day, as she sat next to my bed, telling me about her day and asking me to fight, I left my body and found myself in a beautiful barn with four horses. I could smell the intoxicatingly strong scent of the hay strewn all over the ground. There were four stalls that separated the horses, but they were close enough they could nuzzle each other. There were two next to each other and two across the aisle from those. In the middle of the stalls, an area about the size of a walk-in closet had a few bales of hay I could sit on.

As I watched the horses nuzzle their noses with each other, I began an anguished inner struggle. I knew my family wanted me to heal and come home, but I also knew my mom had been praying that I could die to end my suffering if I was not able to start healing soon. There every day she saw firsthand how much of a struggle it was for me and couldn't stand seeing me in such pain.

I also knew that if I never progressed past this point, I would forever need 24/7 care. That kind of life would be nothing but hell with my independent personality.

As these thoughts floated through my mind, I saw a thick, white rope on the ground and picked it up. It was about a foot long with knots tied every two inches.

At the same time this was happening, I could also see Grandma Dar sitting next to my bed, still talking. My physical eyes were closed, and I appeared to be sleeping.

Inside the barn, I got angry. Like, really mad. As I watched the hospital scene, I started pulling the rope from both sides in anger. I was angry that I was so weak I couldn't even open a bottle of grape juice. I was angry that I was in constant pain and my body felt so foreign. I was angry that I now thought of the hospital as my home and doubted I would ever recover enough to go anywhere else. I missed being home with Matt and spending time with friends. I was angry I'd been forced to suffer when I knew full well God could heal me if He chose to. I wanted more of the rare moments like the days Mom took me to the cafeteria for a Häagen-Dazs bar and a (wheelchair) drive-by of the gift shop.

I wanted a freaking break from this tedium, but I couldn't get one. I had setback after setback. It all felt so helpless.

Pulling on that rope gave me a chance to release some of the pent-up anger and feelings of helplessness. As I started to calm down, I dropped the rope, then walked around the barn, talking to the horses and petting their soft faces.

I think horses are good for mental health because I felt my attitude shift. The worries I felt just a few minutes before became less overpowering.

As this realization hit, I returned to my body having decided to try to appreciate the trials I had been given and find a way to become healthy enough to be released. I knew I needed to put in the effort to strengthen my atrophied limbs when my physical therapist worked with me, even if the only way I could participate was by having a nurse prop me up as I tried not to fall over.

I knew the healing journey would be long, but moving forward, I felt a new push to find something happy in each day.

Chapter 25

Forget Me Not: The Memory Heist I Didn't Sign Up For

As my soul floated through fluffy clouds infused with layers of white light, feeling carefree and unburdened, the Ancient One told me that certain memories were going to be withheld as I recovered. I could experience them now and even learn things here, but I would not remember them once I returned fully to my body.

A deep sadness engulfed me. I didn't want to forget. Every part of me wanted to cling to those moments, to take them with me, to call them forward whenever I needed the reassurance that the Other Side was within my grasp. Each one was beautiful and sacred and part of a greater truth I was only beginning to understand.

As he said this, a burgundy journal with gold writing on the front floated in front of me, a pencil to the left of it. I tried to grasp the journal and pencil, but they floated just beyond my reach no matter how I tried to touch them.

I wanted to plead, to beg, "Please don't take any of my memories from me," but I knew it was not up to me.

I know now that the reason some memories were taken was because it was extremely hard for me to return to my body each time I left. These extra memories made the desire to return "home" too intense. If I could remember all of it, it would break my heart not to be there. The Other Side would become an unhealthy goal. I would not be able to fully live in the present because I would constantly yearn for where I'd been cocooned in love and safety.

The Ancient One told me that when I recovered, I would never again have to deal with the negative effects of ulcerative colitis. I would be healed. I was shown a woman in her thirties with a colostomy bag. The bag floated away, and I was told she was cured. I knew this woman was me, and it gave me hope that I could live a normal life, free of unending hospitalizations, doctor appointments and harsh medications.

Even though my large intestine and appendix had been removed in December, basically "curing" me of ulcerative colitis, my colostomy bag and J-pouch presented many lifelong medical problems. They were not a cure. Did I dare believe what the Ancient One seemed to promise? That I would someday be free from all this?

A J-pouch is like putting a small Band-Aid on a large bleeding cut. You can slow the bleeding, but it doesn't cure the wound. Most prognoses said I would trade an awful set of symptoms for another set of symptoms I hoped would be easier to live with in the long run.

There have been many, many times over the years I have begged God to return my "lost" memories, especially when I have been at a low point or my health has been fragile and I needed that reminder— that I am here for a reason and must keep moving toward the finish line. And even though the memories don't come back, the prayer works. I do remember the big picture, and I do keep working through mortality. But that doesn't mean I'm not eager and excited for the day all these hidden memories return, when my soul slips from my body and I take my final breath and arrive on the Other Side for the last time.

Chapter 26

The Ugly Blue Room: If Walls Could Talk, They'd Complain Too

On Valentine's Day 2000, I was transferred to the rehab area of the hospital, or transitional care unit (TCU) to regain my strength and the muscle I had lost.

My health finally started stabilizing, and everyone's thought process went from waiting for me to die and making funeral arrangements to planning for the next steps in my recovery.

I had spent time on multiple floors and units of the hospital, and this one was by far the worst. I hated rehab and begged my doctor to let me go home. I was the youngest patient by at least fifty-plus years, and it was such a cold, lonely place, with the ugliest shade of turquoise on the walls. I didn't know any of the nurses, and it was hard to keep up with the constant physical therapy and rehab required of me.

My patience grew thin, but instead of crying and giving up, I voiced my frustrations. My fevers were gone, and I felt more like my old independent self.

When Matt visited, I would ask him to hold me. I felt so alone and scared. I needed his comfort. He would lie next to me in my hospital bed and wrap his arms around me. After months of lying alone, surrounded by sterile walls and clinical routines, I was starved for human touch. I had been so deprived of closeness—of simply being held. I missed the feeling of my husband's arms around me more than I had words for. In those brief moments, with his body next to mine, the loneliness lifted just enough for me to breathe again.

Each day, my mom showed up and took me for walks along the sidewalk outside the hospital in my wheelchair, letting the sun warm my pale skin, before wheeling me down to the cafeteria. We ate as I people-watched. I saw pity in the eyes of those watching me. I couldn't blame them. I was skeletal. Patches of my hair were missing. I was hooked up to *all* the IV poles. I looked gaunt and haggard and could only eat a few bites, and I still couldn't even unscrew the lid off a glass juice jar. I had no core strength because I had no core; it had been shredded by so many surgeries.

I weighed seventy-nine pounds now and still required full-time care, but I was determined to get out of there come what may. Each day, I hoped I would wake up, get out of bed, walk on my own, and that my doctor would agree I was progressing well enough to release me from this hellacious prison.

Instead, each day was a repeat of the day before, and though I had taken a moment of hope from the horses on the Other Side, I was once again spiraling into a dark place. It was at this point I gave up and succumbed to the thought that I was not going to get better and my doctor would never release me.

I knew what the Other Side had to offer, and I prayed I could die so I could leave the TCU. Because the worst thing about this stage of my recovery was truly devastating: as my condition had become less critical, I lost the ability to leave my body. I was a constant prisoner to it now.

My atrophied legs felt like Jell-O. To walk at all, I had to use a walker with two people supporting me on either side. I still couldn't sit up by myself, and there was a daunting amount of work to do to get back to my pre-hospital strength.

One day, after my catheter was finally removed, I called a nurse to help me to the bathroom. When she didn't come right away, I decided I could not wait. Desperation took over. I somehow managed to roll sideways and drop to the cold, hard floor. As I tried to stand, my legs buckled and I collapsed to the ground. And that's when I lost control and peed all over myself. I was mortified and started crying hysterically because I didn't have the strength to get up. When my nurse arrived, she couldn't find me because I was on the side of the bed farthest from the door, lying in my puddle of shame, my humiliation as hot as the urine swamping me. I had been in many embarrassing situations during my stay, but this one was at the top of my list.

I thought nothing could compare, but stay tuned. My body managed to pull an even more humiliating stunt that left Matt mortified and questioning why he married me. It was a doozy, quite literally.

I started to doubt I could learn to take care of myself, but I also knew I was withering away in this current hospital ward and needed to break out somehow.

After many conversations with my family, my mom wrote my surgeon a letter asking if he could release me sooner if my family agreed to take over my care at home. He eventually agreed that if they could take on the tasks of my daily care, drive me to rehab three times a week as well as to all my doctor appointments, he would release me to the care of my parents and an in-home healthcare nurse.

Since I fully relied on others for all my basic needs and could not be left alone, I was surprised when my surgeon agreed. I had so many medical supplies to take home that we had to pack a two-shelf wheeled cart twice to take everything down to the car.

As my nurses wheeled me outside, I could smell freedom. It felt intoxicating. I vowed to become healthy enough that I never had to step foot in a hospital again. I had not been inside a car or sat upright for more than a few minutes since December, so every bump on the drive home burned and nauseated me. You need to be proud of me because I did not vomit. I had been given a pillow I was told to hold against my stomach to help alleviate the pain, especially if I coughed. Hugging it helped me arrive home without barfing. At home, a nurse came daily to help change my dressings, check for infection, and teach me how to care for my colostomy bag. One day, as she changed my bag, she casually mentioned that I should sew a pretty cover for it so it would not embarrass my husband if we were intimate. The horrified look my mom gave her was priceless! I thought she would start stuttering. My stomach was still wide open, and I looked like some twisted medical experiment gone wrong, very wrong. Intimacy was the last thing on my mind. I was just trying to get through each day. But there was my mom, wide-eyed, mouth open wide, looking as if my nurse had suggested I run a marathon instead of . . . well, that.

Along with the nurse, my home medical team consisted of my parents and Matt. Still on leave, my dad took on the task of my daily care while my mom and Matt worked.

One of my first memories of being back home was trying to pull my overall straps up over my waist to reattach them after going pee. I lost my grip, and the straps fell down past my waist. I tried to bend forward to pick them up while holding on to the shower door handle, but the door rolled to the left and dragged me sideways. Still clinging to the handle. I slammed into the wall. I didn't have the strength to pull myself up, so I lay there on the bathroom floor, thinking, reasonably, *I have to stay here with my overalls around my ankles until Mom gets home from work.*

I was on the floor long enough that my dad asked timidly through the bathroom door if I needed help.

Well, no. I did not like the prospect of my dad seeing me this way. I still had a shred of dignity left.

At the time, I didn't find it funny that this was the second time I had fallen while trying to use the bathroom. But tragedy plus time equals comedy, and my peeing incidents were comedy gold, pardon the pun. I was eventually able to scoot my back up against a wall into a semi-sitting position, after which I paused to catch my breath. After strategizing how to use every ounce of strength I had left, I slowly worked the overalls up over my legs and, with a series of tiny shuffles and quiet scoots, finally got them over my hips. With my bum covered, I could at least ask my dad to come in and help me stand. Another shining moment of humiliation—but I was so grateful he was there.

Three days a week, my dad took me to physical therapy sessions at a rehab hospital a half hour from my parents' home. I couldn't pull myself up to get into his tall Ford F-150, so he built a wooden step stool for me and kept it inside the passenger door. When it was time to get in, he lifted my feet onto the stool one foot at a time and then lifted my body onto the seat. I leaned into him as he helped me walk to and from the PT sessions since I was still dragging my left foot behind me like an extra in a zombie movie.

We celebrated each success at PT, even if it was something as small as being able to stand on my own for a minute while holding on to the walking bars.

There were many moments where I felt useless, but as I stuck with it, I started having days where I logged more wins than losses. On the days my dad couldn't watch me, I went to work with my mom or Matt so they could babysit me.

I was still very self-conscious about how I looked and wanted to curl up in a ball and disappear when I had to go anywhere other than medical appointments. As my hair continued to fall out and there were only small patches left, my mom took me to a wig store for women going through chemo. We bought a brunette, shoulder-length bob with bangs.

Which I hated passionately. I didn't look like myself in it, it was hot and uncomfortable, and it symbolized surrender. I felt like I was giving in and losing the little bit of myself that was still me. I always loved my long, thick hair, and the wig was fake hair. I never wore it, though I felt bad my mom spent so much money on it. She had such compassion for my struggles and wanted to make things easier for me in any way she could. But the wig was not me.

The one highlight was when Breezi took me shopping for a few hours one weekend. My mom was nervous to let me out of her sight, but as Breezi pulled up in her Honda Civic, my excitement was through the roof. Our first and only stop—Target.

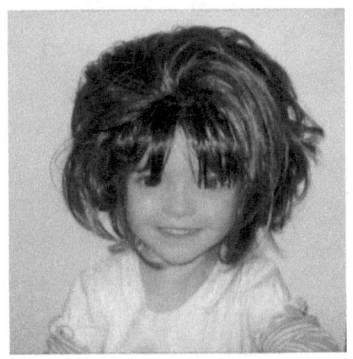

A photo op with the infamous wig, unearthed years later from my hiding place of shame.

As the automatic doors swooshed open, the store's fluorescent lights felt like a spotlight. Breezi entered the store with her beautiful bright-red hair blowing in the wind. I dragged myself behind with missing patches of hair, dressed in my gray, Kmart's kids-department sweats. Breezi gently placed me in an electric scooter, and I gripped the handles like I was in the Indy 500. The motor buzzed to life with a satisfying hum. I pressed the pedal, and the cart lurched forward like a stubborn donkey.

Whoa, I'd forgotten what speed felt like. I was winded from sitting.

As we coasted down the makeup aisle, my cart made a high-pitched, obnoxious *beep beep beep* when I backed up to turn around.

Breezi disappeared around the corner. I heard her scream, "Marco!"

Without missing a beat, I screamed, "Polo!"

A woman peeked up from her station in the clothing department.

"Welcome to our sitcom," I wanted to tell her.

I hit the gas and flew around the corner, searching for Breezi. A small child stood there in awe, as if watching a racecar driver. I gave him a big thumbs up and almost crashed the scooter.

I found Breezi, and we dissolved into laughter interrupted by occasional winces of pain—but it was real. I'd forgotten what laughing in public felt like as I adjusted to being outside a hospital, not hooked up to machines. My face looked like a haunted Victorian child, but I wasn't in a hospital gown. I wasn't intubated. I was surrounded by one-dollar candles and overpriced snacks, shopping with my best friend. I was winning.

"I feel like I escaped something I should not have survived," I whispered.

Breezi went quiet for a minute. "You didn't just escape, you flipped off Harlan the Horrible."

We passed the frozen-treats aisle.

"Add some popsicles to the cart," I said. "I need one for the road."

All too soon, I grew tired. It was time to go back to my parents' house to rest. We had reached a turning point in our chapter of friendship where joy and trauma coexisted. This day, this simple trip with Breezi, made me feel more alive than I had in months. I'd given myself permission to laugh again. To start living again.

Chapter 27

You Again? Because I Just Can't Stay Away

On March 28, I had to go back. I started to have problems breathing and pain whenever I lay on my right side. To my doctors, this sounded suspiciously like pneumonia with a side of pulmonary embolism, or blood clot in my lung.

I didn't realize how bad my PTSD could be until I was wheeled into the ER that day. I tried to calm my rising panic as my doctors approached. I was terrified they would admit me and I would be living at the hospital again.

My worst fears were confirmed.

My oxygen saturation levels had dropped to between 75 percent and 82 percent. They are supposed to be at 100 percent. After an EKG, chest X-rays, a ventilation-perfusion scan to check for pulmonary embolism, an abdominal CT scan, nuclear-medicine imaging, and blood work, I was diagnosed with a pulmonary embolism causing hypoxia (low oxygen in my cells), pneumonia, and tachycardia. My heart rate stubbornly stayed between 140 and 160 beats per minute.

So, crap.

They started IV antibiotics to begin the healing process, and I was released to my parents' care two days later. My relief was so great I would have burst through the doors or danced if my legs could support my weight for two steps.

But they couldn't. My family once again took turns taking care of me as I remained unable to provide for my daily care. I'm sure it was a weird situation for my teenage brothers, but they each showed they cared, even if just by hanging out in my room and listening to their favorite bands with me or taking me for car rides to get out of the house. They were good brothers. I was glad to have them around.

My doctor said as soon as I weighed 110 pounds, I could discuss the next phase of surgeries (Yippee!! *Not*) to remove my colostomy bag and reattach my newly formed J-pouch internally. That felt like an amazing, but impossible, goal. My weight continued to hover between eighty and eighty-two pounds, which was a major concern. My surgeon weighed me every time I saw him, but my body couldn't retain the nutrients necessary to gain weight. I still wore a size 10/12 in children's clothing, and even that was baggy on me. I could see the knobby bones in my knees and arms, and it hurt to sit down because I had no fat on my bottom (plus the tailbone issue). I carried a pillow to sit on at all times. I was so malnourished and anemic, I looked like a walking skeleton with a white surgical glove stretched over it.

Determined to increase my weight, my doctor assigned me a nutritionist. My mom was to feed me two milkshakes a day with small meals every few hours, even during the night. I was cranky, weak, constantly overfull, and it hurt to breathe. There wasn't any room for the milkshakes in my shrunken stomach.

But the strangest part? The only two foods I craved with such a primal intensity it made no sense were McDonald's pancakes with butter and syrup and Grape Crush soda. I had never even liked either of these before. In fact, I couldn't remember the last time I cracked open a can of soda. I joked that all my blood transfusions had changed my DNA and that I craved all of my donor's favorite foods now. Maybe I was now part pancake-loving stranger?

I imagined accidentally meeting my blood donor at McDonald's, both of us reaching for extra syrup packets at the same time. "You too?" they'd say, holding a six-pack of Grape Crush. I'd nod slowly. "Yup, I finally found you."

My family thought it was a weird combination, but they were glad to see me eat anything, so they kept me stocked up on my junk food. We spent a lot of time at lunch buffets, too, where I nibbled like a bird. My stomach had shrunken to a half-cup capacity. Those bites had to be chosen carefully because any more than that and I would get a sharp stabbing pain in my belly.

My mom, knowing I'd been a strict vegetarian since the age of twelve, started blending chicken and hiding it in my food without telling me, trying to bulk me up with protein. Years later, one of my brothers let her secret slip. I was so grossed out I thought he was joking, but my mom reluctantly admitted it.

"Don't worry, though," she said. "You never ate any of it anyway."

Even though I found it hard to eat food, I could chew ice all day. I could not get enough of the crunchy goodness. It didn't hurt my stomach like food did and was cold and refreshing. Here is my favorite recipe from coming out of my ulcerative colitis:

SNACK:

Freeze some water.

Put it through an ice-cruncher machine.

Eat with a spoon.

Repeat.

Chapter 28

Here We Go Again: More Surgeries and Still No VIP Pass

It was my birthday. I was turning twenty-one. The big one. The milestone. The "you're finally legal" celebration that's supposed to come with blurry photos, bad decisions, and enough glitter to ruin your sheets for weeks. Instead, I felt like the soggy contents of my colostomy bag.

I was a week out from my last hospitalization and knew I would not be celebrating like a typical twenty-one-year-old.

I chose to go out to dinner with Matt, my parents, and my brothers to The Mayan—a local Mexican restaurant. It was built like an ancient temple, with actual cliff divers who jumped off an actual cliff into a pool below. *Inside* the restaurant. You could sit at your table in a treehouse setting and watch the show while eating. It was a favorite restaurant of mine (I mean, *cliff divers* and *tacos*. Cliff divers *and* tacos.)

You'd think it'd be hard to be miserable with chips and guac in front of you and men cannonballing from fake cliffs—but I managed just fine. Honestly, they could've set off fireworks and unleashed a mariachi flash mob and I still would've been curled up in my booth, contemplating the cruel ironies of life. It was loud, festive, and full of people living their best lives while I was silently dying in a booth under a fake tree.

I should've been out with Matt. Or with friends. Dancing my face off at a bar, wearing something borderline inappropriate and laughing so hard my stomach hurt—but in a *good* way. I should've been ordering shots with ridiculous names and toasting to adulthood with sticky glasses and bad decisions. Instead, my doctor flat-out told me that alcohol could kill me—not in a "you'll regret it tomorrow" way but in a "you'll literally die" way.

Meanwhile, I watched the people around me live the life I wanted like it was a scene from a rom-com—laughing, pain-free, full of bad decisions and good eyeliner. And here I was, biting my lip so hard I might as well draw blood just to keep the tears at bay.

Pain stabbed through my stomach like it was auditioning for a horror film. I gripped the edge of the table like I was about to be flung off the Tilt-A-Whirl of agony. My mom leaned in, eyes full of concern. "Are you okay?"

I shook my head. Not even a little bit. Not even in a "let's pretend" kind of way.

I closed my eyes for a moment, trying to imagine I wasn't slowly unraveling from the inside out. I barely touched my food. The first dive act was starting, but all I could think was, *I'm not going to make it to the second round.* I asked the waiter to box up my food like a sad little party favor.

A tear escaped. Then another. My body was falling apart, and, now, so was my mascara. Fantastic.

I told my family to stay and watch the show. My oldest brother, Shawn, offered to drive me back to my parents' house. Always my protector, he walked me out, then met me at the restaurant entrance with his car. I was too weak to walk to the parking lot.

Like a defeated gremlin, I curled up in the passenger seat, hugging my knees to my chest. Shawn tried to make small talk, but my body was basically on fire and I couldn't even fake a nod. Instead, I stared blankly out the window, grieving the life I used to have—one where birthdays didn't feel like a cruel joke.

When I got home, I changed into the pajamas of the walking cliché I had become and collapsed into bed. "Happy birthday to me," I muttered, bitterness coating my words like cheap frosting. Honestly, if I'd had the strength, I would have screamed. Loud. Primal. The kind of scream that rattles windows and maybe makes a neighbor call the cops. Because this was So. Damn. Unfair.

And just to twist the knife a little deeper? My mom took pictures on a roll of 35 mm film that night, and the roll was lost. Actual film. Every awkward pose, every forced smile, every excruciating moment— gone. Vanished. No photos. No evidence. Honestly? Good. It was the universe's only mercy that night. Because if I ever saw myself in those moments, I don't know if I could handle it. Some memories are better off buried in the black hole of a Walgreens photo lab.

Remember a few chapters back when I fell off the hospital bed into my own urine like a clumsy ballerina?

Well, not to be outdone, one morning while Matt and I slept, I heard a scream that sounded like a wild, wounded animal. As I opened my eyes, Matt flew off the bed as if he had been launched into the air. He ran toward the bathroom, dry heaving.

This is entirely too early in the morning for whatever is happening here, I thought to myself in my still-sleepy stupor. I had been in the middle of a really good dream I wanted to finish. I looked closer at Matt and realized he was covered in something that looked like . . . Oh, no, it couldn't be!

I sneaked a peek at my colostomy bag, which had torn away from my stomach and drenched us both in hot, smelly bodily waste. Yup, just as I feared. This realization woke me up pretty fast. As Matt leaped into the shower and turned it to the lava-hot setting, I tried to think of a way to get out of bed by myself because I had been unfairly abandoned.

Okay, maybe that's a bit harsh. I would have done the same thing if the roles were reversed.

I thought back to the infamous urine incident and decided to roll off the bed in much the same way, then crawl into the bathroom. I had been waiting my entire life to use the stop, drop, and roll method from elementary school. It was my time to shine! As I gracefully fell to my death, er, I mean the floor, I heard Matt wildly talking to himself. I won't repeat what he said, but he didn't sound like he was excited with his morning wake-up call. Sometimes he is so hard to please. Men, am I right?

I half crawled, half dragged myself into the bathroom as I apologized for being such a gross wife. Matt mumbled something about this being a shit show. Savage, Matt, savage! I immediately broke into maniacal fits of laughter. I am sure Matt thought I was deranged, but all of the pent-up frustration I felt over my inability to take care of myself was released. Matt didn't find any of this amusing and avoided eye contact as he wiped away a few tears he swore were from allergies.

After we both cleaned up and Matt's allergies mysteriously disappeared, I promised to never cover him in my bodily waste again. I kept my fingers crossed behind my back. Don't tell Matt, please.

I came to despise my colostomy bag and everything it represented. What's not to hate about it? Of all the bodily functions no one wants to be made public, this is it: poo container. Of all the organs not to lug around taped to the outside of my body, "rectum" is number one—or number two, actually.

That stupid bag was a steep learning curve, and Matt hugged the edge of the bed and slept with one eye open for weeks.

I learned two important lessons that day.

First, Matt can fly. That was a surprise to both of us.

Second, life can be hard sometimes, but laughter can get us through the worst.

I almost didn't tell this story for obvious reasons: Jealousy. I didn't want anyone to become too envious of Matt. After all, he hit the jackpot when he said, "I do." I mean, I was quite the catch at that point, total dream girl.

Dealing with a disease that involves bodily functions brings a level of vulnerability I wouldn't wish on anyone. It's awkward, messy, and, let's be honest, completely humiliating at times. Honestly, if there was a raffle for illnesses, I would have gladly traded mine for something more glamorous. Something that didn't involve discussing bowel habits like I was narrating a National Geographic documentary.

I could have left out the more vile parts of my story. Trust me—I was tempted. There are some memories that make me cringe so hard I feel it deep in my body—like a shudder that starts in my gut and ripples outward. But I also know that somewhere out there, someone is just as scared as they navigate their own diagnosis. They want to hear the real version. The raw, unfiltered version of what *could* happen. Pretending is actually messier than reality and doesn't help anyone. They need someone to show them that even though life can be scary and downright gross, they are not alone.

Because even though this disease can strip you down to your most vulnerable self, it doesn't get to steal your voice.

And if I have to be the slightly—too—honest, occasional sarcastic trail guide through the land of medical mayhem to prove that, I will.

So, here we are, mess and all.

∾

Over the next few months, I slowly gained muscle strength as I continued physical therapy. I even put on some much-needed weight.

In July, at a regular checkup with my surgeon, I passed the weight test. (He didn't know it, but I had added heavy, smooth river rocks to the pockets of my denim overalls because I was nowhere near 110 pounds, but the point is, I passed!) I felt like I was finally on the road to recovery, though, and I was fed up with wearing a colostomy bag. I wanted to complete my final surgeries and regain some of the life I had lost to my illness and recovery.

Generally, J-pouch surgery is done in three procedures. The first surgery removes the colon and creates an ileostomy. In the second, the rectum is removed, and the ileum is formed into a pouch to replace it and then connected to the anus. The third surgery comes eight to twelve weeks after the second surgery to reverse the ileostomy and reat-tach the small intestine to the pouch. Due to my previous complications and long hospitalization, my surgeries were more complex, the concern over side effects greater than normal.

In July, I had two exploratory surgeries to make sure my small intestine and the J-pouch portion still functioned well enough to be reconnected internally during my final surgery.

I had looked forward to this final surgery since my first surgery in December 1999. I knew it would free me to live a fuller life in the most normal way possible.

My surgery was scheduled for August 2. I was nervous to go back under the knife. My fear of having something drastic go wrong again felt overpowering. It was loud and constant, like a drum beat I couldn't silence. I had already defied death. Why tempt fate? The thought of willingly going under the knife felt like walking straight into a lion's den. It kept me up for hours at night.

I tried to prepare everyone just in case I didn't make it out alive. Morbid, I know. But I had seen how fast life could slip away. How good health could be lost in an instant. I was spiraling fast. I even had professional portraits taken of Matt and me—the ones at Walmart's photo center, with the fake, painted backdrops. Deep down, I was afraid I would die during surgery and these would be our last photos together.

It's strange how preparing for the unknown can make you feel completely in control and powerless at the same time.

The first J-pouch surgery ever performed by any surgeon was in 1976. Before that, people with ulcerative colitis lived with colostomy bags. Before that, people with ulcerative colitis died in horrific pain. Going into this make-me-or-break-me surgery, I felt the time since 1976—just a few years before I was born—was both current-events-recent and ancient-history-old. Mostly, I hoped Dr. Briggs had performed enough of these surgeries to not let me reach "critical" again.

It's a major operation that typically takes between six to ten hours with two to three months to fully recover. But because of the complications during my other operations, my surgeon warned that those "typical" expectations were pretty much complete unknowns for me. He gave me fascinating (scary!) information about possible side effects, including excessive bleeding, the potential risk for lots of kinds of infections, and various ways my body could react adversely to the trauma of yet another abdominal surgery. Also, all my complicated and messy scar tissue made the surgery more risky as well. It was a lot to hear.

I chose to go ahead with the surgery because I couldn't imagine life attached to that stupid colostomy bag. I was twenty-one years old and had my entire life ahead of me. I wanted to live again and not be held back in any way. I hated everything that bag meant and represented.

As I was wheeled into surgery, my entire body shook uncontrollably. I was deathly afraid something would go wrong.

When I woke up in recovery, I was groggy and immediately wanted to know if my unwelcome friend was really gone. I moved the hospital gown away from my abdomen to look.

Just bandaging. This should have brought shouts of hallelujah!

But on the other hand, I was not ready for the amount of exhaustion, nausea, and pain I felt. The weight of my skin and bones was a thousand times too much for what my muscles felt able to move or even lift. The anesthesia was as nauseating, disorienting, and generally nasty feeling as always, except—bonus—it was not working to dull any pain, just to further dull the grogginess in my brain. No, the pain was not dull; it was dazzlingly sharp, hot, and terrible. The skin from my ribs to my hips might as well have been on fire the way it blazed through the brain fog. The moment it eased even barely perceptively, I fell into the mercy of a heavy, dreamless sleep that lasted hours.

I would stay in-patient for at least a few days to closely monitor my condition in case I had an emergency situation that required another surgery.

On day three of recovery, my hematocrit levels, which had been at forty-two post-surgery, dropped to 23.5. This was bad. Blood needs iron to do its bloody job, and hematocrit is a measure of iron levels in the blood. They do not let anyone lower than thirty-eight even donate plasma—the *not*-iron part of the blood. I got blood transfusions yet again, with two units of packed red blood cells—the *very* iron part of the blood—to increase my hematocrit to 33.2.

This hospital stay was different. I was able to better articulate my needs, and I advocated heavily to be released as soon as my doctor felt it was safe. I forgot how loud all the beeping hospital machines were, and knew I would heal faster at home. This time, I didn't complain when my nurse came to help me with my daily hallway walks because I felt one step closer to release.

On day six, I went to the bathroom and used the toilet like an adult human! This was a huge milestone for release. Dr. Briggs declared my J-pouch (his handiwork, of course) a success and allowed me to go home.

Of course, there were complications. Need you even ask?

On August 16, I found blood on my clothes—a lot of blood, coming from my stomach wound (the ostomy). I was readmitted for a few days. The ostomy was the hole in my abdomen wall where the detoured poop exited so the remaining intestinal tissue could heal without having to work that sh—stuff out. Well, mine had somehow developed a new, secondary injury, the source of the midmonth bleeding. This was a short stay, and once the new lesion was chemically cauterized, I was told it should start healing, and they sent me home again.

But again. This is me. The ostomy never really stopped bleeding. Less than a week after I came home, on August 24, I called Mindy, my neighbor across the street, for a ride to the ER because Matt was at work.

I told her, "Every time I cough, my insides bulge out. And there is a blood-clot-looking thing coming out of my stomach wound, and that seems, like, serious. Even to me."

Mindy was very fast in getting me to the hospital.

I had called ahead to let them know I was on my way.

Dr. Elwood met me in the ER, where he ushered Mindy and me into a hospital room reserved and prepped for me.

I lay down and exposed my stomach. I have a pretty high pain tolerance, and a lot of the area around my many incision wounds and scars was still numb from the nerves not being healed. So it didn't hurt very much when the doctor stuck three fingers of his gloved hand right into the stoma to feel around for damage and see how far the injury went.

I glanced over at Mindy, who had a look on her face. I raised my eyebrows questioningly. She darted her eyes at the doctor and tried to whisper, "Hottie."

It wasn't quite as inconspicuous as she hoped. The doctor heard her and jumped a little, eyes wide and face reddening. Laughter involves abdominal muscles. My pain tolerance was higher than my funny tolerance, and I had to bite my lip in order not to laugh.

Dr. Elwood finished his exam without looking at my face, then quickly decided I needed another surgery. There had been very minimal healing of my incision. That meant there was a possibility that my small intestine would come out of my stomach a third time and a very good chance I would develop an infection if it didn't close that night.

During this surgery, fifteen feet of gauze was inserted into the wound to keep my intestine securely inside my abdomen. Over the next few weeks, the wound needed continued cauterizing, and I went to follow-up appointments with my doctor until he felt the threat was over and the gauze could be removed. The day I could take the gauze out fell on a Sunday. I didn't want to wait for a weekday appointment. I wanted it out now!

I tasked my sister-in-law Kate with this deed. She was a vet tech. In my humble opinion, that seemed close enough to a doctor. It was incredible to watch her take it out. She just kept pulling and pulling. It was so long I don't know how it all fit inside my tiny stomach. I thought it was fascinating. My family, not so much. My three brothers scattered like I had lit the house on fire. Matt stood frozen, like he had just witnessed a crime scene. My mom held her hand over her mouth, dry heaving.

It smelled just as you would imagine your insides smell like—rancid, sour, and overwhelmingly like death.

It was the last time my mom allowed her living room couch to be used as an operating table.

With that complication out of the way, I felt like I was finally on the path to recovery. I was hopeful that this twelfth surgery was my final one.

Chapter 29

Grab the Duct Tape: We're Going In

Coming home from my long hospital stay had its challenges, some more overwhelming than others.

While I was in the hospital, Matt took over paying the bills, which had always been my job. A few weeks after my release, I received a letter from our bank that our checking account was overdrawn. As I went through our bills to figure out the cause, I realized that paying bills was not something Matt excelled at. In fact, he admitted he had gone to Wendover with a friend and lost our mortgage payment in a bet. Our mortgage company was starting a foreclosure on our house, and my SUV had been repossessed. Even though I couldn't drive, when the repo company showed up to reclaim the vehicle, I wanted to melt into a puddle of shame and soak into the ground. The repo man (which is not a profession known for tact, kindness, or empathy) looked at me with such pity as I signed the paperwork I thought he might actually cry.

He looked at all eighty-six pounds of me clinging to the doorframe and looking like a medieval plague victim with a few patches of straggly hair, pale skin, sunken cheeks and eye sockets, and said, "Maybe you can get another car down the road if you ever get better."

And then he took my car.

Every day, the mailman delivered another stack of medical bills from my hospital stay—separate charges for each of my four surgeons, the anesthesiologists, and the radiologists' reading fees.

My financial situation felt hopeless. I knew we needed to come up with a plan as fast as possible. I may have been weak, but I could spend my days making phone calls, and that is exactly what I did. I called our mortgage company first. After I explained my medical situation, they agreed to work with us to become current since we'd never missed a payment. Each month, we paid our entire mortgage payment plus 50 percent more for six months until we caught up. I also called every single medical provider my health insurance had not covered and set up monthly payment plans. I was paying so many different billing departments that some agreed to take only five dollars a month until my balance was paid off. The hospital consolidated their separate bills into one payment. My medical bills were close to $300,000. After my health insurance paid their amount, I owed around $20,000, which is still $20,000.

I had page after page after page in a notebook that was nothing but a list of every provider I owed. But my system worked. My spreadsheets, side gigs, and bargain-bin budgeting—it *worked*. A year and a half of scrimping, hustling, and doing mental gymnastics just to keep the lights on, and finally the day came: the last bill.

I wrote that final $141 check like I was signing a peace treaty after a bloody war. It was to Utah Radiology Associates, of course. The final boss. The Darth Vader of billing departments.

They had refused to budge on payments—no flexibility, no compassion. Every time I tried to negotiate, I got a robotic "we'll send you to collections" threat in return. Classy. Real patient-care vibes.

I stood in my kitchen, checkbook in hand, grinning like a maniac. I wanted to do a full-on happy dance, strobe lights and all. And yes, I added a little something in the memo line. Nothing too wild. Just a tiny typo. A harmless Freudian slip.

Utah Radiology Asses.

Oops.

Not petty. Just poetic.

And when I dropped that envelope into the mailbox, I swear I heard a choir of angels. Or maybe it was just my neighbor's wind chimes, but still. That moment felt sacred. It was the end of a long, grueling chapter. I had faced every financial nightmare they could throw at me—nearly lost our house, had my car snatched, watched my credit score flatline—and I still came out on top.

That check was more than a payment. It was a mic drop.

Just like that—after drowning in medical debt, after the stacks of bills that haunted our kitchen counter, after months of scraping by to avoid foreclosure, after watching a tow truck roll away my car like it was taking a piece of my soul—it was over.

Paid.

Done.

Zero balance.

I laughed—a short, stunned little sound at first that grew into something feral and unhinged, the kind of laughter that comes from way too many nights spent crying on the bathroom floor. I covered my mouth, not sure whether I was about to sob or scream. Probably both.

I danced in my kitchen, the laminate floor squeaking under my bare feet. I didn't care. I was spinning. Twirling. Laughing. Crying. *Free.* The chains were off.

"*We're done!*" I shouted to no one in particular.

I flung open the windows. Sunshine poured in as if the universe had waited for this moment too. The air smelled like spring and possibility and hope—the kind of hope that comes with knowing the worst is behind you. For once, I wasn't bracing for the next hit. I wasn't calculating how long we could stretch a tank of gas. I was done losing sleep over the mortgage. I could breathe.

I accomplished something that seemed so impossible. It was a lot of work, but I was proud of the effort we'd put in to settle all the debts and rebuild our credit.

Matt and I celebrated that night in the best way possible—with hot, gooey, cheesy smothered burritos, rice, refried beans, and fried ice cream. After we filled our bellies, we went to a car dealership and upgraded to a vehicle that came to a stop when Matt pushed on the brake pedal. Life was going to improve. I could feel it!

There was one company that just would not work with me—my car loan collection company—unlike the repo man, who, frankly, had better bedside manners. I took a massive hit to my credit for that little venture. Watching my car get hauled away like it had cheated on me was humbling. Oh, they were the real villains in this saga.

The guy called five times a day.

Every. Single. Day.

Morning, midday, just as I sat down to eat, right before bed—like he had a sixth sense for when I might be feeling a shred of peace. His name was Chad. Or maybe Brad. One of those names that sounds like it comes with a Bluetooth headset and an inflated ego.

Chad was from the repo collections agency, and he had zero empathy for the fact that I was recovering from multiple life-threatening surgeries. I explained my situation again and again: I almost died. I was barely able to walk across the room without needing to lie down. I didn't have money. I had medical debt, a mountain of it, and I was holding my body together with sheer willpower and McDonald's pancakes.

His response?

"Well, maybe you should get a job as a hooker. At least then you'd be useful."

Silence.

I blinked.

No. He did not just say that.

My hands shook not from weakness but from rage. From humiliation. From being kicked while down.

This man, this smug voice on the other end of the line, thought it was appropriate to say *that* to a woman who just survived death, who fought to keep her house, who lost her car to his goons.

And for what? A few hundred bucks a month?

So I did what any emotionally fried, sleep-deprived, broke, and freshly pissed-off woman would do: I fought back with what I had.

The next time Chad (or was it Brad?) called, I told him I would send him the amount due. He sounded excited. He would finally reach his quota.

I pulled out my Monopoly set from the closet—yes, the dusty old box with a missing thimble and crumpled board—and crafted my reply like an artist.

Then I took a fat stack of Monopoly money: orange $500s, green $20s, and even a pink $5 for flair. Slid them all into an envelope with a handwritten note.

And wrote:

Dear Chad,

    I have enclosed all of the money I have. You will not get another dime from me. You are a horrible human being. I hope Karma bites your butt.

    Sincerely,

    Heather

I dropped it in the mail and walked away like in a slow-motion movie scene. If I'd had sunglasses, I would've put them on.

It was the first time in months I felt like I had even a shred of control. The repo already happened. The damage to my credit was done. But that day—I got the last word.

And it felt good.

I'd like to think it got intercepted by a secretary who laughed so hard she cried, my power reclaimed, my little middle finger to a system that wanted me to beg.

I may have lost a car.

I may have been sick, broke, and exhausted.

But I *never* lost my fire.

And then, a few days later, my phone rang.

It was him.

I answered my phone, "Well, well, Chad. Hello, there! Did you get my payment?"

"Heather . . . Heather. Really? This is so immature."

His voice dripped with smug disappointment, like a dad scolding a teenager for toilet-papering the neighbor's house.

And all I could think was *Ohhh, it worked.*

The Monopoly money hit a nerve. Good. Maybe next time he'd think twice before suggesting a sick woman consider such desperate measures to pay off a debt.

I smiled into the phone and said, "Chad, don't ever call me again."

Then I hung up.

No more apologies. No more shame. No more explaining myself to people who didn't care if I lived or died—as long as the invoice got paid.

I may have been broke.

But I wasn't powerless.

Chapter 30

Guess Who's Been Keeping Secrets?

After I fully returned to my body and started to heal, I worried that my connection with the Other Side would be cut off, that I would never hear the words of my Spirit Guide again. That has not been the case. In fact, I have become even more aware of the daily miracles in my life.

In the years since my NDEs, I have felt my guide's presence and voice as he whispers to my soul in times of need. I cannot control when this happens, but during major life moments, if I listen closely, I can feel his soothing words.

Many times, my guide will tell me of things that are going to happen in my life before they do, such as meeting a specific person for the first time and even telling me where it is going to happen six months before it does. I receive these messages randomly, which can be frustrating because there are times when I ask for answers to things weighing heavily on my soul and the answers don't come. The Other Side has different priorities than we do, and it does not seem fair!

As I think back on my life, I realize there were important times before I got sick where my guide was present and I just didn't know enough to understand what was happening. I believe he's been with me since birth and he'll be with me for the rest of this life. I am grateful for his guidance and comfort from the Other Side. (Though sometimes I wish he cared more about the things *I* want!)

Chapter 31

More Glitter, Less Guts

Over the next nineteen months, I worked hard to heal and reclaim the life I thought I had lost. My skinny little bird legs regained muscle, and I was able to start walking around the neighborhood each night with Matt.

My hair, which had always been straight, started to grow back again, curly and darker, the missing patches filling in.

I started tolerating foods that had been off-limits for years. I introduced one food a week to make sure I could digest it without pain. The first salad I was able to eat, two years after my J-pouch surgery, was a small bowl of lettuce, a few cherry tomatoes, and creamy buttermilk ranch dressing. I was beyond excited since I thought I might never eat salad again. I had really missed the taste of fresh homegrown tomatoes; crisp, crunchy lettuce; and large amounts of tangy dressing. That little salad was bliss!

One food that will forever remain off-limits, though, is popcorn. Every time I walk into a movie theater and smell the buttery, salty scent of freshly popped popcorn, I feel a pang of loss. It reminds me I will always have side effects and feel a little bit different from those without food restrictions. I usually get over my pity party pretty fast and buy a large cup of ice to chew.

Through trial and error, I found that most foods cause some degree of stomach pain. The only consistently pain-free foods are hard-boiled eggs, avocados, and hard candy. I have learned over the years what works and what doesn't and have come to enjoy meals more than when food felt like the enemy.

Each day as my health continued to improve, I found more of my old self. I learned to see all the miracles that are part of our daily lives, miracles I had not noticed before. The sunrise each morning reminded me of the light at the entrance to heaven. Each time I paused to smell a flower, it felt like a whisper from the Other Side—a gentle reminder of the vibrant greenery I had once moved through so effortlessly, where plants glowed with their own inner light and everything pulsed with peace. I started to enjoy the taste of good food again, a little at a time, and I laughed more because I consciously created joy in my day-to-day interactions.

I spent time planning my future and didn't worry about dying anymore. It was refreshing after being sick for so long and being afraid to think of where I would be in ten or even five years.

During my regular check-ins with Dr. Briggs, he charted my weight and made sure I was healing fully, which I finally was. During one visit, I decided to broach the subject of whether he knew what had happened while I was critical. After he checked my belly scar and sat down to add notes to my chart, I said, "You know that when I was in the hospital, I died, right?"

At these words, his body visibly jerked back, almost as if I'd slapped him. He instantly looked away, avoiding eye contact for the rest of my checkup. He never answered me. Instead, he moved on as if he had not heard me. After that encounter, I was careful to only talk to family and a few close friends about my death and the Other Side. Many, many years passed before I brought it up with anyone else.

Chapter 32

Just Checking Out. Be Right Back!

One day, while watching television by myself, I heard my Spirit Guide tell me my body would not support a healthy pregnancy; when the time was right, adoption was the route to grow our family. I had been so busy healing that pregnancy was the furthest thing from my mind, but I knew what he'd said was true. I had been through too much, and if I wanted to be a mom, I needed to adjust my expectations away from carrying a baby to term.

I started researching and found that fertility significantly decreases after J-pouch surgery, with only 36 percent to 56 percent of women who try to become pregnant after surgery finding success. And with traumatized internal organs, there's usually a higher risk of miscarriage.

I started reading up on adoption agencies and which countries had the best foreign adoption-friendly laws. Guatemala was first on my list. I had taken six years of Spanish in school. I knew I could make sure that any children we adopted remained immersed in the culture of their country of origin while creating traditions in our family. I spent months scanning pictures of all the babies. Unfortunately, the minimum age to adopt was twenty-five, and I was twenty-two. Three years felt devastatingly like a lifetime. I knew we weren't ready to adopt right that minute, but seeing the faces of these sweet babies made me want to become a mom sooner than later.

Before my hospitalization, I had worked at the pediatric clinic with Breezi. I once had a foster care patient who had been abandoned in a park. His foster mom brought him in for medical appointments, and I was so charmed by his adorable personality and curly brown hair that I was pretty much smitten after two appointments. Even when he didn't feel good, he tried to smile at the staff.

I didn't know much about foster care, but I knew I wanted to be a mother above all. I began thinking about how I could fill my arms with these little children until they returned home while I waited to adopt from Guatemala.

I researched foster care, and Matt and I attended an orientation to familiarize ourselves with the process and have our questions answered.

The Winter Olympics were held in Utah in February of 2002. Matt and I spent the entire month taking classes to become foster parents, and missed all the celebrations surrounding this once-in-a-lifetime event, because I felt an internal push to complete the training and paperwork as fast as possible to be ready when the chance to foster came.

Start to finish, the entire process took six weeks. The caseworker who helped us complete our paperwork said that was unusual, but I knew God had a plan, preparing us for what was to come.

Before we started fostering, I wanted one more surgery done—a scar revision to repair some large areas of painful scar tissue and a hernia. I scheduled my thirteenth surgery for March 11, 2002.

The hospital was right up there next to colostomy bags on my list. I had the absolutely rational fear (PTSD) that if I went into the hospital, I might never leave it. So I found a surgical center and a surgeon who agreed to perform the surgery outpatient. Dr. Briggs, who performed my colon removal and almost all J-pouch-related surgeries, was brought in to consult with Dr. Hunt to make sure the surgery was successful.

This surgery went well. It took the eight-inch scar from my rib cage to my pubic bone and moved it down to look more like a Csection scar. I was sent home a few hours later, with two tubes to drain potential infections.

I was unable to take any pain medication after this surgery because it made me so nauseated. This delayed the healing process significantly because pain management is a critical part of recovery. Sleep is crucial to healing, and a body in severe pain can't sleep. After a few days, I was spiking high fevers and shaking uncontrollably. Sure enough, there were multiple pockets of life-threatening infection in my stomach.

As I lay in bed, I felt like I was slipping away again. My mom called the after-hours on-call doctor in a panic. The outpatient center was closed. He suggested I go immediately to the ER, but I was too weak to move. In a last-ditch effort, before going to the hospital, my mom called some church elders and asked them to give me a blessing. The bishop arrived with two elders. As they stood around my bed and placed their hands on my head, the calm feeling I had in my most critical episodes at the hospital returned. It wasn't a promise of ease or painlessness, just a calm sense of knowing what was coming and that I would survive it. They prayed that I would heal. As they spoke, I knew without a doubt that I was going to go critical again, fast, and then, as before, I would leave my body.

After they blessed me, my mom sat next to me on the bed. As the men continued to chat softly with my mom and Matt, the room filled with countless spirits. It was as if the air itself became sacred, with not a single inch of space left untouched by the Other Side.

Tears rolled down my cheek as a deep sense of peace washed over me. I welcomed the moment. I had waited for this. A chance to finally leave my body. In hushed reverence, I whispered to my mom that the spirits were surrounding me, holding me, loving me.

I was ready to go home again.

I felt that familiar exquisite love again. And with that, my soul slowly lifted out of my body, hovering about three feet above my bed, weightless and free.

I watched as Matt spoke with the elders and my amazing, sweet mom kept a close eye on me, and I basked in the love I had missed so much since I began healing enough to stay mortal. Pure, intense, radiant peace washed over me. I felt so relieved to be out of my body and once again in this warm, familiar cocoon of light. Being out of my body was like going home after a long journey and being wrapped in the loving arms of my family. Nothing else mattered. No pain, no burdens, just love.

As I hovered above my body, I somehow knew this was the last time I would leave like this, the last time to so freely touch the edges of heaven. I felt like I was saying goodbye to my time on the Other Side. Even as I savored this moment of heaven, I simultaneously felt an emptiness and sorrow, grieving the loss of it. I felt like I stood at the edge of a cliff, whispering farewell to the wind. The steep rocks below made it impossible to cross. I could feel the pull of the Other Side. I could reach for it—but I could not touch it.

It was like saying goodbye to part of myself—a final, devastating goodbye.

Unfortunately and fortunately, my spirit did stay in the room and reunited with my body. I knew from that point on that I would be healed and no longer need surgeries.

After the elders and bishop left, the on-call doctor called back telling me to immediately return to the ER for surgery to remove the extensive pockets of infection. As Matt and Mom helped me get ready, a staple popped out of the incision on my stomach. All the infection built up inside gushed onto my bathroom floor, and my fever dropped.

I stared in complete amazement and knew I had been granted a gift and the healing process would now fully happen without another surgery.

I let the doctor know about the spontaneous clearing of the infection and told him I would not be needing to go to the ER. We agreed I would go in immediately if things changed or if the fever returned.

From that point forward, although I was still very weak, I started to heal. It was not the beginning of the end, it was the end of the end. My full, deep recovery was not immediate, but I was finally leaving a chapter of my life behind. Each day, I became stronger and stronger and started planning my future without fear of surgery or death.

Chapter 33

The Little One Who Changed Everything

One ancient Chinese proverb says, "An invisible red thread connects those who are destined to meet regardless of time, place, or circumstance. The thread may stretch or tangle, but it will never break."

On March 31, 2002, our foster care license was approved and went active. We were finally able to indicate that we were open to respite, shelter, foster care and adoption/legal risk cases.

Respite placements are kids already in foster homes who need to be temporarily placed in another home for many reasons, from the caregiver having some sort of crisis or getting sick to the family leaving town when the child needs to stay near their birth family. Shelter-care kids are emergency placements—children who've just come into care, or come abruptly, and the placement workers are looking for extended family who can pass a background check and step in to take the children while the parents work on the issues that landed their kids in care. Foster care cases are children who are waiting for extended family to pass a background check to take the kids or who are generally not going toward the route of adoption. And adoption/legal risk cases are when the child's case might go to adoption at some point, but it's not guaranteed.

Whenever a young child is considered legal-risk and adoption can occur if family is not available, a committee of DCFS workers chooses three to four families with home studies that match the needs of the child. They hold staffing meetings to choose the best family to support and foster the child in their home. A resource family consultant is assigned to become the foster parents' support person.

This consultant represented our home study in this meeting and then offered support when we had a placement.

Our first placement—a fourteen-month-old baby girl named Victoria (Tori)—arrived late in the evening on April 23, 2002. Her mother had asked that she be placed in a home that could adopt her, knowing she wasn't in a position to raise her.

We had no idea she was coming.

Tori's caseworker, Zendina, was brand new and clearly overwhelmed. She had forgotten to call us earlier in the day to let us know we'd been chosen by the placement committee. She didn't call until she was practically in our driveway. I didn't even have time to run to the store for diapers. I didn't have baby formula. I didn't even have an ETA.

When I opened the door, Zendina stood there, stiff and expressionless, awkwardly holding a chubby little bald baby in urine-soaked yellow pajamas. Her diaper hadn't been changed in hours. The baby clutched a sticky bottle of chocolate milk, her cheeks blotchy from crying. Her blue eyes, wide and confused, darted around like she was trying to understand what was happening—where she was, who we were, why everything smelled so unfamiliar.

There was no warmth in Zendina's face. No sadness. No tenderness. No acknowledgment of the heartbreaking gravity of this handoff.

She handed a plastic grocery sack to Matt. Inside were three old, mismatched outfits and four diapers. That was all.

I reached for Tori as Zendina offered a rushed explanation. She handed me a thin, purple three-ring binder with limited medical records, said she'd be in touch, and left just as quickly as she came.

The moment the door closed, everything shifted.

Matt and I were excited, yes—but more than that, we were heartbroken. This tiny girl had just lost everything familiar. She didn't know us. She didn't know where she was. Her little face crumpled, and she began to sob.

I wrapped her in my arms and held her close. She was shaking. We took her upstairs, cleaned her up, changed her diaper, and dressed her in a white onesie I had tucked away just in case. Then I wrapped her in the softest blanket we had and carried her into her new bedroom.

There, I sat in the rocking chair and held her tight. Her cries eventually softened as I rocked gently back and forth, whispering and humming lullabies against her tear-stained cheek. My voice shaky with emotion, I sang to her, barely above a whisper.

Eventually, she fell asleep. In one of the purest, loveliest moments of my life, I knew right then and there that I would do everything I could to protect and love her. She had been through a lot in her short little life. I knew she needed to warm up to us, to feel safe before she could fully let down her guard, and I was beyond willing to give her all she needed to get there.

As soon as Tori arrived, my body, which up to this point had not been able to lift over ten pounds, was suddenly able to carry this precious child and give her every ounce of love she needed. Another miracle. This ball of chunkiness and pure bliss weighed twenty-five pounds. I was careful when I lifted her, and I never tore the scars that were still very much healing.

We spent hours playing in her bedroom and outside as she got used to her new environment. I had decorated her room in pink-and-white gingham wallpaper with a border of vintage baby dresses. It was my favorite room in our house. Tori and I took daily walks to the nearby park and played outside on her swing and in her sandbox in our large backyard. The extended family adored her. She was spoiled with attention, snuggles, and love from all directions. Everyone who met her fell in love instantly. But no one more than me.

Tori taught me the true meaning of love.

Being her mama—even if only for a season—was the greatest reward of my life.

For six wonderful months, this precious baby girl filled our home with endless laughter and love. When I close my eyes now, I can still hear her beautiful little laugh echoing down the hallway. I can hear that laugh—oh, that laugh—and the way she said Mama, drawing out the last *a*. I can see her taking her first steps across the living room and the look of accomplishment on her face. Her look of surprise when she lost her balance and tipped over. I can see all the funny faces she used to make. She had a silly, playful personality.

Her eyes lit up whenever we visited a shoe store. This girl loved shoes almost as much as I do. I would catch her in my closet, trying on my high heels, attempting to walk as she stumbled around, a huge grin on her beautiful face.

One of her favorite games was to dump her bowl of noodles on her head when she was full—and then fall into a fit of giggles, completely amused with herself.

Being her mama was pure joy—the kind that makes your chest ache in the best possible way.

She was my little ham.

My first baby.

My greatest *gift*.

I truly believe we healed each other. She thrived with us, and my broken body healed at such a fast rate I almost forgot I had been so sick. I had never been happier.

On October 15, the DCFS judge awarded custody of Tori to her grandparents, who lived in another state. They'd learned she was in custody in Utah and asked to adopt her. Since that time, we had been visiting with her grandparents as the case moved through the legal process of deciding who would raise this little one.

Family is always first, and since there was nothing in their background preventing them from raising her, she returned to her birth family the next day.

I will never forget her caseworker showing up as our closest family and friends took turns saying goodbye to our sweet girl. We spent the morning packing all her clothing and toys so she would have some of her daily comforts. Zendina made me empty half of her belongings on the sidewalk because she said I packed too much.

It was overwhelming for me to decide what was most important to send with her when all I wanted to do was spend the next, final precious moments holding my baby and giving her a lifetime of love.

As I placed her into the car seat and told her I would always love her to the moon and back, a dam of such intense loss burst inside my heart. It was easily as painful as anything I felt in the hospital. I grieved from inside my bones and soul and wanted nothing but to hold her one more time. As the car drove away, I wanted to run after it, grab my baby, and never let her go. The ache in my chest was so deep it hurt to breathe. She had been my lifeline.

Now she was gone.

As I stood in the middle of the street, watching the car turn the corner and disappear, I felt dead inside. I was just a shell, watching the world move on without me.

The fresh loss was almost out of my control. My pain was so heavy I lost my appetite, and over the next few weeks, I lost ten pounds. My arms ached to hold my baby, and I worried that she would think I had abandoned her. Foster care at that time did not encourage interaction between foster parents and birth families after children returned home. I worried she would wake up scared at night and her family wouldn't know how to help her. She had to have her favorite plaid blanket and two teddy bears to fall asleep. Would she have severe trauma from being moved to another state and into a new environment without warning? I didn't know if I would ever know she was okay, and I felt like I had died inside.

The world has a way of blessing us with miracles sometimes, though, and this was no exception. A few months after Tori went to live with her grandparents, her family reached out to Matt and me with an update and some pictures, even though such interactions were discouraged. The photos were adorable. Her face was ever-so-slightly thinner, more like a little girl and less like a baby.

Since then, we have developed a close relationship, and I have been able to watch my sweet girl grow up while continuing to be a part of her life. She is one of my greatest joys, then and now. I am endlessly grateful to her family for allowing me this gift. Knowing she has been loved and cared for helped me to move forward. I know in my heart that even though I would have moved mountains to have been her forever mama, she was placed exactly where she needed to be to give her the experiences necessary for her life story. And I still get to be part of it.

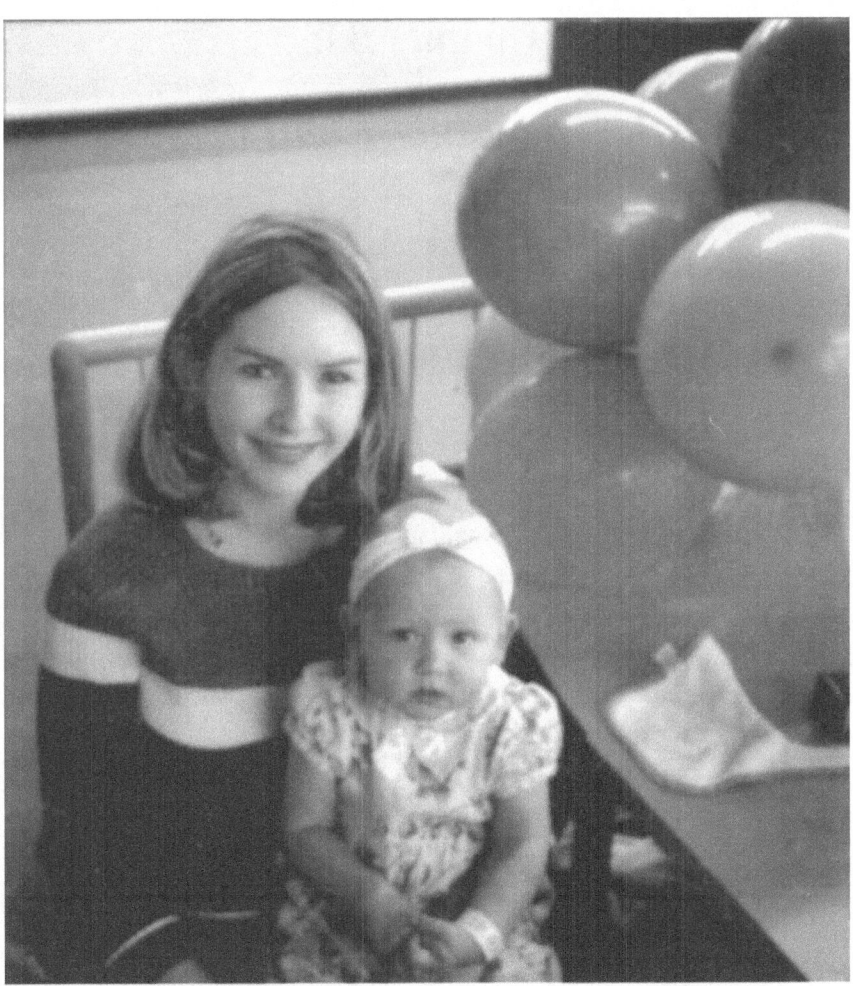

My first week as a new mama.

Chapter 34

The Adventure Continues

On October 17, the day after my beloved baby girl left, we received a call from another caseworker. They had a two-week-old baby boy named Alejandro who needed a temporary foster family for a month or two, until he could reunify with his two-year-old brother and father. He was baby number eight born to his mother. Due to her drug use during each of her pregnancies, DCFS stepped in and took custody of each new substance-exposed infant at the hospital, the babies placed with extended family. For years, because she refused to complete treatment, with each new baby, the judge had moved to terminate her parental rights.

I told the caseworker we would foster the baby and then told Matt that Alejandro seemed like a consolation prize since they felt bad we had lost our little girl. He was grieving as well and said that having the distraction would be good for us. I decided to pour my energy into this newborn while helping his dad prepare for his arrival. I could try to heal from my loss at the same time.

I bought tiny outfits and baby care supplies and went to pick him up from the hospital with my mom since Matt was at work. It was bizarre to walk into a hospital with an empty car seat and walk out with a live baby I had met only ten minutes before.

He was a tiny bundle of love with a head full of soft black hair. When he fussed from drug withdrawals, I wrapped him in blankets fresh from the warm dryer, then rocked him in the rocking chair.

I made a scrapbook for his dad with all the pictures I took at the hospital and during his time with us so he could know about the first few months of his son's life. I brought him to his weekly supervised visits at the DCFS office so I could interact with his dad and make sure he had the information and skills to parent his son.

Knowing this baby was temporary helped me to start to heal from the loss of Tori and not get so attached to this little one because I knew his time with us was limited.

Three weeks after his arrival, on Halloween, as my mom and I bought baby clothes at Mervyn's for this little guy, I received a call from our placement caseworker. She told me the placement committee was considering two possibilities: a six-week-old baby girl or a twenty-two-month-old baby boy who was classified as a legal-risk case. I had never taken our name off the adoption list, but I also didn't expect a call so soon.

The voice of my guide was back, as always, whispering over my right shoulder. I heard him say that we would be chosen to foster the little boy and that the baby girl would not go toward adoption with us but would be placed with an older sibling.

I definitely did not want to go through the grief of a failed adoption again, but I told the worker to consider us for both, fully knowing that the baby girl was not ours. I later found out she was indeed placed with an older sister, and I was happy they would be raised together.

On November 7, I received a call from our worker that the placement committee had chosen us to foster the little boy. I had been told his first name was Treyvon (Trey), that he was biracial, and nothing else except that I could come to pick him up at the Christmas Box House shelter.

A fierce storm brewed outside. Wind lashed against the car. I drove down the freeway, gripping the steering wheel and dodging the garbage blowing across the road. Alejandro, snuggled in his car seat, a blanket wrapped around him to keep him warm, slept soundly. I was babysitting my friend's two-year-old for the day, so he joined us in the adventure as well.

My first sight of this little boy made my heart swell. He was bundled in a dark-blue, puffy winter coat; a blue-and-white plaid fleece hat; and tiny white K-Swiss tennis shoes. A caseworker helped me get everyone loaded back into the SUV, and we made the drive home. Trey was quiet for most of the ride as he took in his surroundings.

When we got home, I gently removed his winter gear, finally getting my first good look at him. This skinny little twenty-two-month-old had a head full of gorgeous curly blond hair and hazel eyes that stopped me dead in my tracks.

My heart skipped a beat. This was the little boy from my hospital vision.

This was the little boy who came with the little girl and the old man. It felt as though some long, invisible thread that connected us eons before this moment had just been tugged. Sweet baby boy was born on December 26, 2000, one year and six days after I was admitted to the hospital. I hadn't thought of that child for months, but here he was, stealing my heart and blowing my mind, my beautiful boy.

Not officially, though. Not yet. We were considered a legal-risk home for him, meaning the ultimate goal was for him to return to live with his mom, but if that wasn't attainable and his extended family couldn't adopt him, we would be given the option to adopt.

We went from having one sleepy, cuddly newborn to a household with a very active toddler who was quite the handful and wouldn't sleep at night. So I didn't ask for any more placements for a minute and spent my time acclimating to being the foster mom of a rambunctious boy.

A few weeks after Trey arrived, our newborn foster baby, Alejandro, was reunited with his brother and dad. It was a beautiful reunion, and I knew his dad would love and protect him and his older brother. He appreciated the scrapbook I made of Alejandro's time with us and asked a lot of questions about his needs and daily care. Again, I felt confident he would be the dad his son needed.

Since Trey's current plan was reunification with his mom, he saw her weekly. I would drop him off for their three-hour visits, then stay in the area—shopping or visiting the nearby library to stock up on books since it was a forty-five-minute drive back home. However, one day, thirteen months after Trey's arrival, when I dropped him off for a visit with his mother, I felt an urgency to get back home, unpack all my newborn baby boy clothing and supplies, and get them ready before picking him up from his visit. It wasn't just a thought but a sense of urgency, a knowing.

The feeling was intense, like a voice telling me over and over that a baby boy was coming and I needed to be ready. I gripped the steering wheel and blinked hard, trying to shake the feeling. But it only grew stronger—an invisible pressure wrapping around me with every passing mile. I glanced at the clock. Traffic was thick. I thought to myself, *This is bordering on the point of lunacy, so maybe keep this to yourself.*

And still that voice repeated inside my head, quiet but insistent: He's coming. A baby boy.

By the time I reached my driveway, I was buzzing with anticipation. I went straight to the baby supply closet and threw open the doors, pulling out the bassinet, setting it up, and wiping it down. My hands moved quickly as I grabbed tiny onesies, socks, and outfits to wash, the scent of Dreft laundry soap filling the air. I moved on to the car seat next, checking the straps and clicking the buckle into place. My hands shook a little—not from fear but from adrenaline. Anticipation.

Although I had felt my guide, the Ancient One, many times since being released from the hospital, especially when I got the call for Trey, this was profoundly different, with such an intensity attached to it that I couldn't ignore the message that came with it.

It was as if the veil between the two worlds had thinned for a moment—just enough to hear, to *know* without question.

As I moved through the nursery, I felt a warmth in the room that had not been there before—not heat, exactly, but a presence. Like someone stood just behind my shoulder, guiding me as I prepared for the baby.

The sense of urgency turned to peace the way a thunderstorm turns to rain. Quieting, calming.

When the phone rang, cutting through the quiet, I wasn't surprised—I felt recognition. It was the call the urgency told me would come—a call about a newborn baby boy to foster.

This communication with my guide, giving me a sneak peek of what was yet to happen, was one of the strongest ever outside the hospital.

Tears welled in my eyes. I felt like I stood in the sun again after a long winter.

I knew at that moment I was not just hearing something divine; I was *part* of it.

It felt amazing and validating.

This new little guy was severely drug exposed, with the highest drug levels the hospital ever recorded at birth. I spent the first two months of his life learning to care for him in the NICU of the same hospital I had so much history with. I visited daily to train on his complex medical needs and bond with him while Matt and my family took care of Trey at home.

It was hard to walk through the doors every day and not hold my breath. The smells of the alcohol swabs and the cafeteria's hamburgers and over-steamed broccoli topped by the stench of cleaning supplies nauseated me. And the constant beeping of the machines was hard to listen to without wanting to scream. When I got in my car to leave the training, I felt like I had escaped prison. Milo was finally released to our family from the NICU on New Year's Eve 2003.

I rang in the new year getting to know this tiny little boy who had fought so hard to live.

For the next twenty months, we worked closely with his parents and their Native American Ute tribe to try and safely reunite him with his parents. His tribe did not believe in adoption by non-native families, and I was told they would continue with reunification efforts until he was eighteen years old, even if his mom never got clean.

He *was* sent home to them and then returned to us six months later for a short time before reunifying again. (Years later, after he left, I got an update that he was with his dad and other siblings and doing well. This knowledge gave me permission to stop worrying about him as his dad was much healthier than his mother).

As Trey, who we had nicknamed Buddy, continued to have visits with his mom, I felt it was important to build a relationship with her. I'm glad I did. I grew to love her and cheer her on when she achieved a goal and grieve for her when she struggled to meet the caseworkers' and court's expectations and timelines.

When a child is in foster care, the court strives for reunification with the birth family or for adoption. It gives a specific time to achieve either goal. For a child under five years of age, less time is allotted since children need stability and should not sit in limbo for years, waiting for a decision while they bond with their current caregivers.

I sat outside the courtroom before the DCFS case reviews with his mom as we waited for court to begin. She talked to her caseworker and her mom about how excited she would be if she had custody returned, and she dreamed aloud that she could be the mom he needed. It was bittersweet to hear. On the one hand, I wanted her to have the opportunity to parent, but I also wanted to make sure Trey had a successful, safe life no matter who raised him. I had to put my thoughts aside and know that what happened was meant to be and I couldn't control the outcome.

Every day, I prayed his mom would know she was loved by our family, that she would gain the skills to take care of her very active little boy, and that she would know we wanted to support her through this process. Ultimately, a year and a half after Trey came into our lives, his case went to trial, and I was subpoenaed to testify.

When the day came, I sat in the sterile courtroom with fluorescent lights. Even now, the memories remain fresh in my mind. I hated every minute of my time on the stand. I wanted to throw up from the anxiety. My palms sweated and my heart pounded.

"Can you please speak louder so the courtroom can hear you?" the judge asked. I wanted to shrink into my seat and hide. I hated that the system had forced me into this role.

I wanted the room to know that Trey's mom really did love her son. I wanted them to see how her eyes lit up when I brought him to visit her. I wanted them to *know* her as a person, not as just another case on their court docket.

I truly loved Trey's mom. Watching her sitting next to her attorney, I knew she was scared. I wanted to take away her hurt, her pain.

In the end, after testimony from the caseworker and other evidence was presented, the judge changed the goal to adoption.

As I watched his mom and her mother sob at the finality of the ruling, my heart broke for them. I knew this day had splintered his birth family.

I left the courtroom with a lump in my throat the size of a fist. I wanted to run after his mom and wrap her in a hug. I wanted to tell her I was so sorry this was happening to her. At that moment, though, I was the enemy, part of the source of her pain—the very pain I wanted to take away.

Instead, I walked to my car in a daze. The dam holding back my tears burst. The sobs came. Deep and gut-wrenching, they rattled my entire body.

And at that moment, all I could think about was Trey's mom. I wanted her to know, *needed* her to know, that he was safe, that her baby was loved and cared for and she wouldn't be erased from his life.

Because I remembered. I remembered how it felt when Tori left. And not knowing had nearly crushed me. I did not want her to go through that same darkness. She deserved to know Trey, to watch him grow up.

Trey had a "goodbye visit" with his mom where she was expected to say goodbye, knowing this would be the last time she ever saw him.

I was not okay with this. I couldn't imagine the magnitude of grief she must have felt that day as she prepared for his arrival. As she checked her camera for new film to capture his beautiful face one last time. As she tried to cover her tear-stained face with makeup. As she put on a happy smile when we arrived. I will never know her most intimate thoughts that day, but seeing the pain in her eyes as she gave Trey a final hug brought me back to the day Tori left. I am sure she wanted to chase after my car. To grab her baby boy. To never let go, just as when I watched my sweet girl leave with Zendina.

I told Trey's mom we wanted to have an open adoption, but I don't know if she believed I would follow through. I knew the more love Trey had in his life, the more it benefitted him. I wanted him to know where he came from and that although he was adopted, he was very much loved and wanted by his mom and extended family as well as by us, his adoptive family.

On April 27, 2004, Matt and I adopted Trey and finally, officially, named him Isaac, keeping his original middle name of Noah to honor the name his mom chose for him.

As we stood before the judge with our extended family and the adoption was granted, so many conflicting emotions tore through my mind. I celebrated becoming a mother while another mother, who I sincerely loved, mourned her loss. I wanted to hug her tight and tell her it would be okay.

Over time, something incredible happened, something I couldn't have imagined on that fateful day in the courtroom.

I was able to develop a very close, deeply meaningful relationship with Isaac's birth mom. It didn't happen overnight. Trust takes time. But slowly, we built a friendship. We had an open-door policy where she could spend time in our home and continue to bond with beautiful, happy little Isaac. She read him books, played with him, and laughed with him. She held him in her arms, memorizing his scent—Baby Magic lotion. It wasn't about shared DNA or legal documents. It was about love. She became part of our family in every way that mattered.

I have had the rare and humbling gift of witnessing her rebuild her life, one single brick at a time.

And in the years after the adoption, I had the honor of standing by her side during some of the most profound moments of her life. I was there when she gave birth to her daughter. Later on, I helped welcome her son into this world. Both times, I watched, fully in awe as these sweet little souls entered this world. I don't think she will ever know how much those moments meant to me.

I am so proud of the mom she has become. Every single day, she shows up for her kids with love and purpose. Her children are happy, healthy, and cherished. They celebrate each holiday together, decorating gingerbread houses and sugar cookies in matching Christmas pajamas. She plans birthday parties with cake, family, and trampoline parks. She takes them to summer county fairs to ride Ferris wheels and roller coasters. She attends school field trips so her kids know she is always there for them, and she works hard to provide a stable and welcoming home. And her children are thriving. They are experiencing the life I know she wanted for Isaac.

My son looks so much like his birth mother that sometimes it stops me in my tracks. The shape of his forehead. The curve of his lashes. It's *her*. She's right there. Living in his beautiful face. The parts of her that I see in him feel like soft reminders of where he came from.

When I look at him, I see a story.

I see survival. I see grace. I see her.

Watching her become the mother she is today is one of the most healing parts of my own journey.

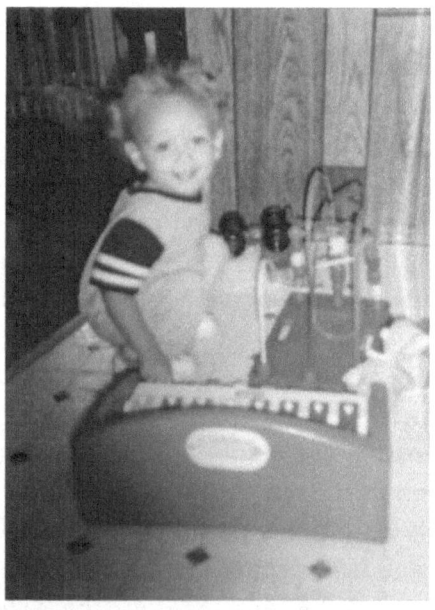

Talk about a déjà-vu moment, when I first met my son.

Chapter 35

The Long-Awaited Meeting

Over the next year after we adopted Isaac, many children passed through our home. I often wondered if the little girl who came to my hospital bed would find her way to us as my son had.

During this time, we had another failed adoption. It was devastating for me, especially as her birth parents were not safe and she should never have been sent home. It was a terrible case where the system completely failed this little girl and her father was later sent to prison for sexual abuse. It made me sick to my stomach.

I had come to know and feel my guide's energy by this point as he had been a continual presence in my life since my hospitalization. When I was alone and it was quiet, I spoke out loud, like I was praying, and asked my guide if my little girl was out there, if I would still be given the opportunity to be her mother.

One day as I drove home from visiting my grandfather, it was quiet, and I asked again. From behind my shoulder, my guide whispered to my soul that she was not yet ready to join our family but would come when the time was right.

I figured she was either not born yet or was (hopefully) safe wherever she was. It calmed me to finally receive an answer, and I thanked my guide. And I quit asking where she was, choosing to have faith that she would come when she was meant to.

Over the years, I've learned that God's timing is not ours and that no amount of pushing and begging can speed it up.

On the morning of June 14, 2005, I woke up with an unshakable certainty. Today was the day. A quiet, knowing voice, the voice of the Ancient One, stirred deep within my soul. It whispered, "Prepare for your daughter." *My* daughter! It started as a feeling, a hunch, a subtle shift in the air around me, the knowledge that I would meet my daughter that day. As morning turned to afternoon, the energy grew—stronger, heavier, buzzing. I could feel a pulsating energy around me, surrounding my heart. I *knew* this feeling. It was a feeling I had only known a few times. Life-altering times. Moments when my world flipped on its axis. When heaven seemed to brush against Earth.

I felt grounded in this beautiful, surreal calm. It was as if my soul had already seen what was coming. It simply waited for the rest of me to catch up.

I felt my daughter near.

I knew, just knew, that by the end of the day, everything would change.

I pictured myself holding an adorable baby swaddled in her blanket. Getting reacquainted with her after years apart. I felt my love for her increasing, and I felt whole again. I had boundless energy as I gathered my baby girl supplies and readied her room. I giggled in delight as I placed the tiny pink dresses in her closet. As Isaac played nearby, I watched in awe, knowing he would also be reuniting with the soul who had been his companion as they watched over me in the hospital. Would they recognize each other in their earthly bodies? The thought made my heart swell with love and anticipation.

Later that afternoon, right around 3:30 p.m., the phone rang.

It was our DCFS resource family consultant. Right as I heard her voice, I knew. This was it.

She told me Matt and I had been chosen by the adoption committee to foster a baby girl—she was eleven weeks old.

For a minute, I couldn't breathe. Tears filled my eyes as I struggled to maintain my composure. My voice cracked as I tried to talk.

It was finally happening. The moment I had felt so strongly about that morning was here, unfolding in real time, that sacred buzz of energy announcing her arrival so accurate.

I immediately called Matt at work. As soon as he answered, I blurted, "A baby girl is coming to our home today." We had been waiting years for our family to be complete, and he was as excited as I was that this case might lead to adoption. This case held the promise of permanence.

It felt surreal, joyful, divine.

In that moment, I knew that every detour, every trial, every tear had led us here. To her.

When I picked Mannix up from her foster family, I couldn't help but laugh a little. She had patches of fuzzy orange hair, intense gray eyes, and rough, red chubby cheeks. Adorable in a "chaos-muppet" kind of way, she was a petite eleven pounds and still fit into zero- to three-month clothing.

Our family fell instantly in love.

Pure light, she radiated joy and sweetness with every little coo, every little laugh.

We nicknamed her Boogie Woogie because as soon as she heard music, her little body bounced with excitement. It wasn't just that she liked music. She felt it. All of it. Profoundly and deeply within her soul. Like it spoke to her. If she heard sad music, her lips quivered and she let out this soul-crushing wail. It was as if she understood music as a language in a way most had forgotten.

She was such a happy, curious, alert baby, her bright eyes soaking in the world around her. She was fascinated with Isaac, especially his curly hair. She grabbed it in her hands and pulled as hard as she could. She was his shadow, scooting after him wherever he went.

Over the next few months, her features changed. Her hair, once fiery orange, lightened to a soft, sunny blonde. When she turned five months old, her eyes—the big expressive windows to her soul—finally settled on the most beautiful shade of hazel green speckled with gold and mischief.

I *knew* without a doubt that this was the little girl who had spent time in my hospital room, the one who was with me when my spirit was between this world and the next.

Watching her grow, it was like my soul recognized her before my arms ever did.

Each week, I brought Mannix to the DCFS office for a one-hour visit with her parents. I'd sit in the lobby, Mannix in her car seat, diaper bag packed with bottles and fresh diapers. Isaac usually found a toy and a kid his age to play with.

Once, on a rainy day, her dad Dave arrived fifteen minutes late, holding his umbrella, hair and clothing drenched. His car had broken down on the drive over, and he had walked—in the rainstorm—the rest of the way to the office. The moment he saw her, his eyes lit up like a Christmas tree. He adored her.

At each visit, I brought pictures to give her parents a glimpse into her daily life. They asked questions about Mannix while also slipping in questions about my family. They needed to know she was safe and adored by our family. Dave asked if she still slept with her arms above her head like she did as a newborn. Her mom, Sarah, wanted to know if she reacted to music, offering the names of a few songs she listened to while pregnant.

They held her close, reading her favorite book, *Love You Forever*, by Robert Munsch. They fed her bottles while staring into her eyes with a depth of love that took my breath away. They were gentle, devoted, and deeply present during those short sixty minutes.

I supported them, encouraging their efforts. We were getting to know each other on a deeper level and developing a bond.

But after a few months, something shifted. I felt it before anyone said it out loud. There was a quiet sadness in the mother's eyes, an uncertainty. Her hands shook when she snapped Mannix's onesie after a diaper change. She looked lost in thought.

One afternoon, I walked into the lobby with Mannix as usual. Matt had Isaac for the day so it was just us girls. Sarah stood near the visiting room alone, her expression unreadable.

"Can we talk in an empty room while Mannix is with her dad?" she asked, her voice cautious.

I nodded.

I handed Mannix to Dave, who took her to another room to feed her a bottle.

We sat on a worn, brown leather couch that had been witness to many families' tears and joys over the years.

"Can I tell you something important?" she said.

"Of course, anything," I replied.

"I need you to know something." Her voice was stronger as she spoke.

"Mannix is my greatest gift. I wanted—still want—to raise her. Something happened when I was pregnant with her."

I waited for her to continue, curious about what had happened. So many thoughts ran through my head of what it might be.

"When I was pregnant, I saw a spiritual medium," she continued. "The woman looked me straight in the eye and told me I would not be the one to raise my daughter . . . but that I would *choose* the one who would."

She paused, hands shaky, eyes filled with tears.

"At the time, I didn't know if I believed her. Not really, until I met you. The first time I saw you with her, I just . . . I knew it was you. You were the one."

I immediately felt the calm presence of the Ancient One in the room. I went quiet for a minute, letting the words sink in. How do you respond to such a powerful revelation?

"It's been hard," she continued, her eyes downcast. "I have struggled with what Mannix will think of me when she grows up. Will she struggle with why I didn't raise her? Will she . . . hate me? Will she be angry that her father and I couldn't give her a safe, stable life she deserved—and that she ended up in foster care because of that?"

Then she looked at me again, eyes searching, full of something deeper than hope—fear maybe?

"You have an open adoption with Isaac's mom, right?" she quietly asked.

"Yes." I nodded. "She is still a very important part of his life. She is family now."

She squeezed her hands together so tightly her knuckles turned white. She looked like she was building up the courage to ask her next question.

"Would that be possible with Mannix? With us, if we cannot complete our case plan?"

The weight of her question was enormous. I knew it took all her courage to ask.

I took a breath, my heart full.

I looked into her eyes. I wanted her to feel, not just hear, every word I spoke.

"Yes," I said without hesitation. "Absolutely. You and her dad will always have a place in her life—and in ours. If you do decide that adoption is the best route, I will honor that choice with all my heart. If she returns to you, if reunification becomes possible . . . I will be there every step of the way as well. I want you to succeed."

Her lips trembled slightly. The tension in her shoulders disappeared.

The bravery it took for her to consider this was beyond herself. My heart wept for the position she was in. I tried to imagine what I would do if the roles were reversed—if I had to make the impossible decision between holding on to my child or giving her a different kind of life. Just that thought brought me back to losing Tori and the unimaginable grief that racked my soul.

"I just want her to know she is loved. I have loved her from the moment I knew she existed," she softly replied.

I could see how much she struggled, every fiber of her being wrapped in love, fear, and uncertainty. As much as I wanted to comfort her, I knew the best thing I could do was step back and allow her to make this decision without my influence.

"Please talk with Mannix's dad and caseworker. Sleep on it. Weigh the pros and cons. I don't want you to make a rash decision and regret it later," I told her.

She nodded, blinking back tears, and pulled me close. I hugged her back, hoping she felt all the love I had for her. Neither of us had dry eyes by this point.

It is hard to put that moment into words. I knew deep down that Mannix would eventually become my daughter, but I was also always very careful to never think ahead and plan a future with her. I didn't want to jinx anything. Also, I really felt a deep love for her parents and rooted for them to be able to parent her as well.

A few weeks later, I got the call.

Mannix's parents had decided to relinquish their rights, paving the way for Matt and me to adopt her.

I sat quietly for a long time after I hung up the phone. That moment was bittersweet in a way I still feel deep in my chest. I promised myself that day that I would always honor her birth family. I would honor their roots. As I held this precious infant in my arms, the scent of her baby shampoo strongly lingering as I kissed the top of her head, I whispered all my hopes and dreams for her future. "You are immensely loved, my little one." I cooed over and over as I rocked her to sleep.

Even with the weight of everything that led us here, I was filled with excitement.

I was going to be a mom—*her* mom, this beautiful, bright-eyed little girl, the one who made every day magical for me.

Together with Mannix's parents and caseworker, we sat down to make an adoption plan. Matt had also spent a lot of time with Mannix's parents and believed that maintaining that connection was best for everyone. We talked about Isaac's open adoption and his relationship with his birth mother—how his face lit up whenever she visited and the unmistakable love that flowed between them. We couldn't move forward without giving Mannix that same gift. She deserved to grow up knowing where she came from. We promised to make sure she always would.

In the years since I saw the two children at the foot of my bed in my hospital room, Matt and I had spoken about the "coincidences" we'd experienced when Isaac and now Mannix came into our lives. I am pretty levelheaded in my daily life. Matt said that when I told him I knew these two children were meant to be raised by us, he was fully on board. We talked about how their visits must have been their way of preparing us for their arrival.

I always attended each court date when Mannix's case was reviewed, and I was present when my little one's parents relinquished their rights, paving the way for Matt and me to adopt their baby girl.

I will never forget the deep anguish etched into their faces as they signed the termination papers in front of the judge, on separate days, heavy with grief. My heart ached deeply for both of them. Sarah's hands trembled as she reached for the pen. Her eyes were swollen and red from hours of crying. I watched her fight an invisible battle as she struggled to steady her breathing. Was she thinking of the day she welcomed her child into this world? The moment she first held her in her arms? As she signed the papers, I imagined her soul screaming inside, screaming for the unimaginable loss she felt. I don't know how she had the strength to sign those papers.

When court ended, I walked outside with Sarah, who turned to me with unspeakable pain in her eyes.

"Go celebrate," she said softly, her voice ragged from crying. She tried to smile. "This is a celebration for you. You have a new daughter."

I was stunned. In the middle of her heartbreak, she was thinking of me and my future with her child. How could I celebrate anything after witnessing something so profoundly devastating? Once again, tears stung my eyes. I wrapped her in my arms, pouring all my love and gratitude into her heart. Holding her close to me, I whispered how much I loved her, how important she was to me and Mannix.

What do you say to someone who just gave you the gift of becoming a mom to their child? There are no words.

The day Mannix's dad relinquished his rights was a stormy, overcast day. As we walked into court together, he tried to stay composed, but that moment shattered him. Deep sobs racked his body. They seemed to come from the center of his soul. I had witnessed this kind of grief twice before—sitting in the courtroom with Isaac's mother and then with Mannix's mother as their worlds collapsed around them. And now, here I was again, watching history repeat itself in the most gut-wrenching way. It was almost more than I could handle.

Dave sat at the courtroom table, pen in hand.

"Are you sure you want to do this?" the judge asked. "It is legally binding."

He didn't answer right away. He put his pen down. He took heavy breaths. I could see his chest rising and falling. The room was silent. I looked away. I didn't want to intrude on his grief. I felt responsible for it.

When he finally opened his eyes, there was a look I'll never forget, a hollow sadness. It settled deep into his soul. Without another word, he signed the papers, looking utterly gutted, the kind of sorrow you don't recover from. It lingers in your daily life. Some days it hits harder than others. It reshapes you as a person. There will forever be *before* and *after*.

When court ended, we stepped into the hallway. Too heavy with emotion, no one spoke. The weight of what just happened hung over us like a heavy fog.

He glanced outside and let out a long sigh. His car was parked on the street, its headlights shining brightly. He had left them on in his rush to escape the pouring rain.

"Are you kidding me?" he muttered.

His car battery would most certainly be dead.

It was the kind of insult life throws at you when you are already at your lowest—as if losing his daughter was not enough. Now he couldn't even drive away, couldn't escape. Couldn't do anything but sit in that miserable, unbearable moment with his shattered heart.

I offered to help. I even offered to drive him home. The weight of the day was heavy on him as his shoulders sagged.

We walked toward a court guard. "Do you have jumper cables?" he asked.

The guard gave him a small nod and asked him to follow him. Before he walked away, he gave me a hug, a sob escaping from deep within him. "Please let my daughter know I did this *for* her, not *to* her."

My heart ached for him and for all the pain both Mannix's parents felt.

I walked to the car in silence, dazed. As I pulled out of the underground parking, I caught a glance of Dave with the security guard, the hood of his car propped open.

My sorrow for the man who had just signed his rights away only to be met with a dead battery was too much. The dam I had held back finally burst. Heart-shattering sobs filled the car.

I gripped the wheel tighter. Today did not feel like a win.

As I prepared to become Mannix's mother forever, I knew I had witnessed the most heartbreaking chapter in someone else's stories.

As we let friends and family know we would be adopting again, everyone was so happy for us, but they didn't see the other side of this equation. Both my children suffered a loss not recognized in adoption nearly enough. I vowed to keep Mannix's birth family close so she could grow up with their loving influence.

On February 23, 2006, our family of three stood before the judge, again surrounded by extended loved ones, and became a family of four as we adopted our daughter, who we named Sienna Noelle.

I am profoundly thankful to both my children's parents for the unimaginable trust they placed in me to raise their babies. I witnessed their grief firsthand—raw and unfiltered. That pain is etched in my soul. I will carry it with me until my last breath. It is part of me. I am humbled by the unselfish sacrifices they made on behalf of their children. I know every Mother's Day and Father's Day has to feel like a kick in the gut, a constant reminder of what they have lost.

As every parent knows, it is not an easy job to raise children, and during the harder parts of parenting, I thought back to the many times these two little souls visited my hospital room, stood at the bottom of the bed, and watched me quietly with their wise eyes, almost as if they were keeping me safe. I remembered the love and peace I felt, and I know they were sent to me all those years before to give me a chance to know them in spirit form before they were born.

Whenever I have been at my lowest, trying to be the best mother I can but feeling like I am failing, I remember that God gave me the gift of knowing of their existence pre-birth. Maybe He did this to make it easier when times were hardest, when I questioned my ability to be the parent they needed. I remembered I was meant to be a mother to these two souls He entrusted me with. This thought gave me the strength I needed to rally and do my best to parent my children because it was not an accident that I became their mom. There is a plan, and things happen as they are meant to in this life. Sometimes I just need to let go of the need to feel some control, and just breathe and keep moving forward.

I always hope that when my children look back on their childhood, they will know I always loved them. I prayed every day for them for many years before they were ever born. I fought to give them the best life possible. I cherish every happy memory we have created together throughout the years. Every hug, every bedtime story, every scraped knee. I am endlessly grateful that my children chose me to be their mama.

Many times over the years, I have been asked if I am sad I was never able to experience pregnancy and give birth to my children.

My answer is always no.

My children came to me as they were meant to. I can't imagine it unfolding any other way. They were written into my heart long before I held them in my arms. I believe they have been entrusted to me in this life, however brief it may be in the grand scheme of things. I hope they know how deeply they are loved.

This journey has filled our home—and my heart—with laughter, love, and lessons from the twenty-five incredible children who came to us through foster care and adoption. Being their mother, whether for a season or a lifetime, I couldn't ask for anything more.

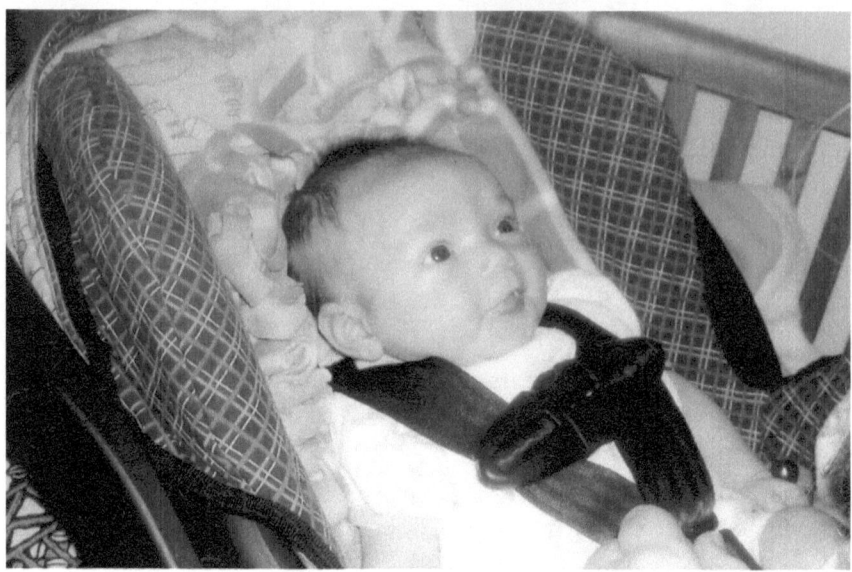

Hello again, baby girl. I've been waiting a long time for you.

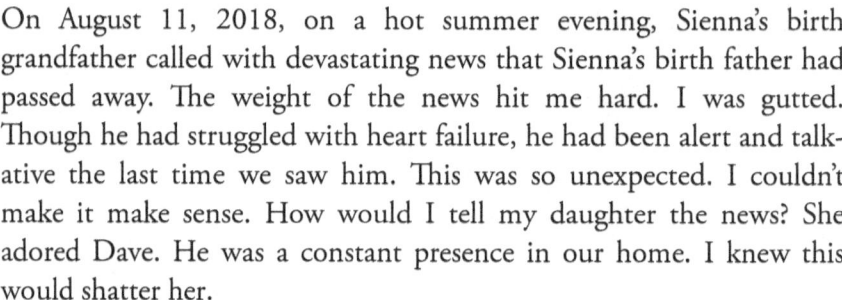

On August 11, 2018, on a hot summer evening, Sienna's birth grandfather called with devastating news that Sienna's birth father had passed away. The weight of the news hit me hard. I was gutted. Though he had struggled with heart failure, he had been alert and talkative the last time we saw him. This was so unexpected. I couldn't make it make sense. How would I tell my daughter the news? She adored Dave. He was a constant presence in our home. I knew this would shatter her.

After I hung up, the phone rang again. This time, it was Sarah. She had heard the news and was already on her way to our house. Sienna was at the neighborhood pool, swimming with a friend. I quickly gathered her and brought her home. When we walked through the door, I cradled her against me, searching for the right words, my voice breaking with grief. As I told her, she collapsed against me into gut-wrenching sobs—the sound of her pain nearly tore me in two.

Sarah arrived soon after. Though she and Dave were no longer in a relationship, she still cared deeply about him. Without a word, she wrapped us both in her embrace, offering quiet comfort. Together, we went to the backyard, where the stillness of the night wrapped around us and the moon cast a soft glow across the yard. The world seemed to pause as she held her only child. It became a sacred space for Sienna to grieve—surrounded by the love of both her moms.

The loss of Dave was undeniable. Sienna hadn't just lost someone in her life—she had lost a part of herself. He was there the moment she entered the world, witnessing her first breath. He was her history, her steady presence, someone who loved her with every ounce of his being. I wished I could shield her from the depth of that pain. Dave is deeply missed. I think of him often, knowing he's still watching over his girl, guiding her from above.

I want to take a moment to honor and acknowledge the birth parents of my children. I will always carry deep gratitude for the part they played in shaping the beautiful souls I now get to call my own. I recognize that my children's story didn't begin with me and I will always hold that truth with love and respect.

These children were entrusted to me to raise during our time together on this earth. They are part of me now, just as they are forever connected to the families who brought them into the world. I do not discount that they have a second set of parents who love them deeply. These children are shared by us both—two families forever bound by love. We are all woven into their story, and I honor that sacred bond every day.

Chapter 36

Keys, Chaos, and Divine Timing

In 2006, Matt and I decided to sell our home. We didn't need such a big house, and I wanted to downsize. We had an offer the first day it was listed, and the realtor promised to find us another home in the neighborhood so Isaac could stay at his school and we could stay close to my parents, who also lived in our neighborhood.

Our realtor failed to find us another home, and I was a nervous wreck, overwhelmed with uncertainty. Matt and I grew increasingly worried about our living situation to the point where we nearly canceled the sale. There were no houses available where we wanted to stay. The pressure weighed heavily on us.

Driving to an appointment one day, I felt my guide whisper for me to sign the closing papers: a neighbor would approach us with a house we could live in, and, most importantly, we would be okay.

I went home and told Matt that my guide had reassured me—a house would be ready for us and it would all fall into place. He knew me well enough to understand that I do not make decisions lightly, without research or reason. Trusting both my instincts and the messages I received, he believed me when I said it was going to be okay to move forward.

I signed the papers with faith that we would be protected and asked the buyers to do a one-month rent back while we searched for another home, which they agreed to.

Shortly after we signed the closing documents, my next-door neighbor knocked on my door. He had heard we needed a place to live until a house became available in the neighborhood. He had just bought a house one street over he could rent to us if we were interested. We were, and that decision became one of the richest blessings in our lives.

The people who lived in this new cul-de-sac became like family. We made countless memories throughout the years. My children had a neighborhood full of friends to grow up with, and I was able to make friends with people who supported and loved me through all the good and bad as we raised our children together.

My kids still talk about those magical summer nights when fire pits blazed in the middle of the cul-de-sac and chairs lined up in a circle like old friends. The adults gathered under the stars, laughing and sharing stories, while the kids ran through the yards playing night games, their laughter echoing through the warm night air. They lived for those days—the giant blow-up water slide, the splash of the pool, running from house to house for snacks while playing with American Girl dolls, riding bikes, and playing basketball in the street. And Halloween—oh, it was the best. The kids piled into the back of a pickup, bouncing around in their costumes and searching for the houses with full-sized candy bars. Later, we all gathered at the designated party house to fill our bellies with soups, appetizers, and laughter. These nights felt like magic, equal parts mischief and community, wrapped in the glow of porch lights and pumpkin lanterns.

Those friendships remained long after many of us moved away. The smell of a bonfire always transports me back to those golden days and brings a beautiful sense of nostalgia, like a whisper from the past reminding me of sweet moments.

After living in this house for four years, we started looking to buy a home within walking distance of our much-loved cul-de-sac. We hoped a house would become available on this street but didn't have any luck.

In March 2010, my realtor asked us to tour a house one street over.

As I walked inside, I *knew* this was our house. It was in rough shape, and my realtor tried to talk me out of it. It had been vacant for eight months and had gone into foreclosure. The roof had flooded over the front-door area, and the walls inside the living room had been replaced with just drywall, patching, and no primer or paint. In the basement, wires hung from the ceiling, and the walls and floors remained unfinished. It could have made a great haunted house.

The kitchen had dark-green countertops, and a sunflower wallpaper border lined the yellow walls. The upstairs bathroom tub had flooded, and mold had grown under the flooring. In fact, for being only eight years old, the entire house was a total gut job. But as I walked through it, I could see it—my kids tearing into presents on Christmas morning next to a brightly lit Christmas tree; their laughter echoing as they played on the swing set I planned to build in the back-yard; summer barbecues with friends and family; and the comfort of being able to walk to my parents' house just ten doors down. This house had potential, and I knew we could make it our home.

Shortly after we submitted the offer, I had a dream where I stood in a hallway with doors on either side stretching endlessly. I walked into the first room on my right and saw my grandmother, who had been with me during my NDEs. She sat confidently at the head of a large, dark-wood, oval table with countless men in business suits filling every seat.

My guide was with me and told me that Grandma had made it possible for us to buy this home.

I believe this is true.

There had been a few times during the process that we didn't think it was going to work out, and we had to come up with a lot more money for a down payment than we were initially quoted. But what I felt the first time I walked through the house was meaningful, so once again, I decided to just have faith.

Finally, we received word that the loan documents were complete and ready to sign. Even better, we got an amazing deal since the home had a previous VA loan. Over the next month, while still living in our cul-de-sac, we remodeled the entire house with the help of family and a handyman friend.

We turned this broken house into a home where our family could thrive.

It was our plan to live there for two years or less and then sell it when a bigger house became available so we could have a larger kitchen and living room to entertain guests.

Life doesn't always turn out the way we expect, and those plans slipped away as this little home became our sanctuary during the harder times that came into our lives. Now, I can't imagine living anywhere else. Even though the kitchen is smaller than I would like, the sweet aroma of banana bread still drifts through the house, wrapping me in warmth and comfort. My kitchen is still productive and cozy. Every day I am thankful for the opportunity to live in such a beautiful area, surrounded by nature, hiking trails and wildlife, and neighbors that can't be beat.

Chapter 37

Alexa, Play "Single Ladies"

In September 2012, Matt and I celebrated our fifteen-year anniversary.

A few weeks later, I jolted awake in the middle of the night, shaken by a vivid nightmare that Matt was having an affair. It felt so real. Tears freely flowed down my cheeks, my crying eventually waking him up. Through choked words, I told him about my dream.

"I would never do that," he reassured as he pulled me close. We both eventually drifted back to sleep again.

The first week of December, I grabbed the mail, like any other day. As I opened his credit card statement, I learned that my dream was not wrong. It had been a foreshadowing. The credit card charges were for items and places I did not recognize, for things that were obviously not for Matt's family.

I was destroyed. Gutted. Betrayed.

As I packed Matt's clothing and my brother changed the front door locks of our house, I could not stop crying. I could not stop crying for stretches of time I can't even remember correctly now. Matt was out of town that weekend for what he *said* was a work event, which gave me time to sit in silence while my kids spent some time at my parents' house.

I asked my guide to please let me know if I was making the right decision. I knew deep in my heart that I was, but this was so new. I'd never been married to someone I *knew* was cheating. Was it *really* the best choice? Maybe I was failing my children by divorcing their dad, but I knew I needed to be strong as I moved forward, to keep their lives as stable as possible. I also knew I deserved better.

I was scared and anxious about how I would handle being a single mom. It had never been on my list of things I thought I would do (you know, like ulcerative colitis). I didn't know if I had the strength to make it work. I had already been through so many kinds of physical and emotional pain, and now I was experiencing betrayal, and with it, a brand-new kind of grief.

In the following days, I put dinner in a slow cooker so my kids had a nice warm meal, but my appetite was gone. I had to choke down a piece of banana bread or a few bites of soup and force myself to drink a glass of water every day. My mouth was so dry I couldn't swallow. It felt like I had eaten an entire bag of cotton balls. It was the holiday season, and friends were dropping off treats, but my usual cravings for anything sweet were gone. The sight of food nauseated me.

My heart felt like it had been split in half. I tried my best to keep it together while my kids were with me, but as soon as they went to school, I used that quiet time to try to make sense of the mess I was in. I ugly cried, sobbing for hours. Every night after I put my kids to bed, I sat on the floor of my bedroom closet, put a pillow over my face to muffle the noise, and screamed until my throat hurt. I *may* have called Breezi late one night as I cut all of Matt's underwear into tiny pieces with scissors. I'll admit I was not at my best.

One day, as I sat in silence, my guide clearly told me that divorce was the correct choice and that it needed to happen now. He also told me that people would be placed in my life as I started this journey, to help me. I would be protected every step of the way.

A complete sense of peace engulfed me at these words. My guide gave me the push I needed to set everything in motion. Just as he promised, incredible miracles unfolded. When money was sparse, something unexpected happened, always at the last minute, and I would be able to pay my bills. I had been praying one day to find a way to pay my monthly mortgage. I told God I was $1,000 short and had no clue how to come up with the money by the due date. Christmas was in a few weeks, and I felt like a failure. I heard a knock on my front door. When I opened it, no one was there, but I found an envelope with $1,000 in cash.

As I held that envelope and wept in gratitude, I knew we were being watched over. Even though it was not going to be an easy battle, I was strong and would find a way to pay my mortgage and provide for my kids.

I connected with people who were able to give me the help or information I needed right when I needed it, including a divorce support group for my kids and me. And I found an incredible divorce attorney who has been my greatest support, fighting hard to keep me and my kids safe and financially stable.

Four months after my separation from Matt, I found a new job working in district court with offenders who were court ordered to complete therapy. This job allowed me to keep my house and move toward giving my kids the life they deserved. A kind neighbor volunteered to watch my kids for a half hour each morning before school so I could arrive at work on time. And I was able to stagger my hours so I could wait at the bus stop to greet my kids every day. We walked home together while each told me about their day. Nights were reserved for dinner, homework, and playing outside until bedtime.

We started rebuilding our life and regaining that missing laughter. It was a simple time I sometimes miss so much.

Eight and a half months after our separation, my divorce was finalized. I was granted full custody, and Matt and his new wife, who he married three days after the divorce was finalized, moved four hours away with her children.

Divorce and single parenting have by far been one of the hardest things I have ever done, but the incredible people who have become my closest friends have stayed by my side, supporting me every step of the way, especially when I doubted I could make it work.

My parents, who still live ten houses away, have been very involved in helping me and my children. They make sure we know we are loved and supported. When my kids were still in school, my mom bought them school clothes, shoes, and supplies each year, lessening my worry about where that money would come from. My kids took many vacations with my parents each year while I worked, and I am forever grateful for their continual presence in our lives.

I always remind myself of the quote "So far, you've survived 100 percent of your worst days." I can look back on those years now, which at the time seemed insurmountable, and find joy in so many memories. My adversities help me appreciate what I have now because I worked so hard to get to this point.

Chapter 38

Vacationing with My Guide

In 2021, when Sienna was fifteen, we decided to take a spring-break road trip to celebrate our birthdays, which fall in March and April.

Isaac had graduated and moved out, and I thought it would be fun to do a girls' trip to Glenwood Springs, Colorado. Three days before we left, I had an ominous feeling that there would be an accident while we drove. I knew I needed to pay extra close attention during the six-hour drive. The mountains that stretch over Utah and Colorado have some of the best scenery but some of the worst statistics for car crashes anywhere in the country. The roads and highways frequently have heavy traffic, and that, combined with the steep inclines and sharp turns in the curving topography, means the driving is fun but risky. I am terrible with directions to begin with, and I had never taken a long road trip where I was a solo driver, so that made me nervous.

Before we left, I said a silent prayer to keep us safe and protected during our drive.

I was glad I did that. Six miles from mile marker 116 and our destination, a huge silver Lexus SUV directly to the left of us (driven by an inexperienced nineteen-year-old girl) moved abruptly into our lane. As the car pulled within inches of us, its front bumper clipped the back of a flatbed trailer attached to a semi. The Lexus became airborne in front of our car before I could process what was happening.

As my eyes watched what my brain had not yet registered, I felt our car glide into an opening in the other lane, as if someone else was steering. I pulled to the side of I-70 without being hit. Until that point, the freeway had been busy, so the fact that I had an open space in the right-hand lane was a miracle in itself. The SUV flew from right to left, spinning through the air in front of us, parts of it spraying everywhere, and landed on the other side of the busy freeway. It finally settled on its passenger side, blocking multiple lanes. Through another big miracle, the driver missed hitting any vehicles on that side of the freeway.

As Sienna and I called 911 and ran across the freeway to help extricate the driver from her vehicle, another group of travelers joined us. They happened to be police officers training for disasters just like this and had the tools to remove her from her overturned vehicle and stop the bleeding from her head wound. They were able to stabilize her until the ambulance arrived.

After my adrenaline wore off, I mentally replayed what had happened. If I had been traveling even five seconds faster, she would have crushed our car, instantly killing Sienna and me.

I felt so thankful I had listened to the voice sent to warn me. I had consciously and mindfully avoided large pockets of traffic throughout the entire trip because, by this point in my life, my guide had been 100 percent correct in his predictions. His guidance saved our lives that day. Traffic averaged speeds of eighty to ninety miles per hour on that stretch of highway. If the young girl had flown to her right instead of left, she would have landed in the Colorado River, which was about fifteen feet off that side of the freeway.

Many miracles happened that day. The right people were put in this girl's path at the right time, ultimately saving her life. After the paramedics transported her to the nearest hospital, Sienna and I made our way back to our car parked on the other side of the freeway. We had to run across lanes of traffic. My heart pounded. I was too rattled to drive.

I kept thinking about the mother of this young girl getting *the call* that her daughter was in a critical accident. Did she drop the phone and scream? Did she have someone who could drive her to the hospital? Was she alone? What would I have done if I received that call for one of my children? I imagined her world tilting. These thoughts were scary and intrusive. I couldn't stop thinking that this could have been one of my children.

I turned to Sienna, my body still filled with adrenaline. "Maybe you don't need your driver's license after all. I can drive you around forever. I couldn't handle losing you."

Sienna was shaken up, but she was still a teenager who wanted her freedom. "Mommm . . . that's not fair," she bellowed. "I'll be careful. I *am* a good driver."

"You've only driven in the church parking lot while I half covered my eyes and clung to the door like it was a life raft. Promise me you will always drive under the speed limit and always be careful. I don't ever want to get a phone call like the mother of that girl," I begged her.

She looked over at me and nodded. "Always."

We agreed on a compromise that she could start driver's ed that fall.

"I love you to the moon and back," I whispered.

As we drove away, still shaken, I thanked my guide for protecting us from tragedy.

Our first day was spent at Glenwood Caverns Adventure Park with a gondola ride to the top of the mountain, where the park is located. I thought right away this would be the highlight of our trip, and we did have a great time that day, flying over the canyon in the giant swing, touring the caves, and riding the alpine coaster. But the best was yet to come.

The next day, we headed to Iron Mountain Hot Springs, right next to the Colorado River. There are multiple pools, from icy to scalding, all full of minerals. I was back in my element.

As I sat in the warm mineral pool, I closed my eyes and listened to the soft music playing throughout the resort. Suddenly, I felt my guide nearby. Together, we sat in silence for a few moments, savoring the serene beauty around us and the gentle sound of the water lapping against the side of the pool's edge. After about five minutes, I felt his whispers of knowledge, telling me I would soon begin a new job. He went on to describe it in detail: I would work in the legal field in an office where I'd find fulfillment in helping others. He told me exactly how much I would make per hour and that my new boss wouldn't offer health insurance so I would need to purchase it through the Marketplace. I was also told that the job would be close to my neighborhood, with the option to work remotely at times. I wouldn't have to search for this job. It would come via word of mouth, and I would know the person who told me about it.

My guide told me to enjoy my vacation and not worry. He said that when I got back to Utah, I could prepare to leave my job and transition to the new one.

Just a little supernatural glimpse of my future.

After returning home, for the next four weeks, I waited, making sure I was completely caught up at my current job. I wanted to leave an empty to-do list for my successor. I was calm as I waited, but I did wonder each day which person would introduce me to the job. Would it be someone I casually started a conversation with in a grocery store? Would it be a work colleague? A friend? It was fun to imagine. I told my mom all the details so we could compare them when the job arrived.

During the first week of May, as I conversed with a friend, she mentioned she had a friend who was hiring for a paralegal position. The office was two minutes from my house. She asked if I could send the owner of the law firm my résumé.

I sent it that night, and the friend called me for an interview that week. As I spoke with my prospective employer and he told me about the job, it felt like he had seen the list my guide gave me as he stated word for word what I had been told, including the exact dollar amount my guide told me I would earn. When he said the best part of my job would be helping people, I felt a sense of déjà vu. Since he was a smaller firm, he said, he could not offer health insurance. I left the interview *knowing* I would be offered the job. He said he would be in touch within the week.

That night, I had a random conversation with a neighbor. He introduced me to an insurance agent who helped me secure insurance from the Marketplace website for Sienna and me. I gave my two weeks' notice two days later, then waited for my job offer.

Those next two days were a lesson in faith as I waited for the phone to ring. They stretched on in an almost holy stillness—like the air before a storm, almost electric. I went about my days with a quiet sort of reverence, in a daze, doing laundry and cooking dinner for my kids, all while I listened for my phone to ring. I knew it would, my faith never wavering.

I checked my phone not out of worry but out of readiness.

And then it did.

I was participating in a family meeting on Zoom with my DCFS team and the birth family we were working with. COVID had shut down all in-person meetings. The ding of a phone notification caught my attention. A quick glance at my texts showed *the one*. It had finally arrived. Hallelujah! Gentle relief washed over me as I read the message. I never doubted the offer would come. This was another moment of divine orchestration. I was exactly where I was meant to be in this life, guided every step of the way.

The offer had originally been sent to my email but landed in spam, which I never check, My heart raced as I slyly opened the email on my phone, pretending to be fully engaged in the meeting. I scanned the subject line, then clicked on it. There it was—my job offer. My eyes darted through the bullet points. Just as my guide promised, they were all there. Every single one.

I never doubted my guide with this one. He had been more specific than ever, but it still felt surreal. I was reading the details that had been whispered to me the month before. I couldn't wait for the meeting to end to tell my mom. I immediately sent her a text. "I GOT IT! I GOT THE JOB!"

Her reply was immediate. "I knew you would. Congratulations! Let's celebrate tonight."

I tried to keep a professional face for my Zoom buddies, but I am sure more than one wondered at my sudden happiness.

When my meeting ended, I logged off, took a deep breath, called my soon-to-be boss, and accepted the job offer.

I was calm and collected during the phone call, enveloped in a hug of inner peace. This was the divine confirmation, the knowing I had waited for.

I had worked at my last job for a total of ten years and was emotionally burned out from dealing with abused children. It hurt my heart to be exposed to the depravity. I knew I had helped, but my capacity for maintaining my sanity was dwindling. For my own mental health, this new job was a bright step in the right direction in so many ways. I no longer had to wake up at 4:30 a.m. to get ready for work. My 1.5-hour daily work commute changed to four minutes. This gave me more time to spend with family and friends and tremendously less-ened my stress load.

This new job wasn't just a paycheck; it was the beginning of a better life.

Each time I hear the whispers of my guide, I regain a few moments of my time in the hospital when I was so easily able to leave my body and spend time in a realm whose primary function was spreading love and healing.

I always welcome these visits and know I have a lifetime for my guide to teach and lead me.

Chapter 39

New Guts, Who Dis?

Although I am relatively healthy now, I still have many, many side effects from the surgeries and medications used to keep me alive. I have lived with pain a large majority of the time since my illness almost killed me.

When the complications become severe and during the most painful times, I question why I was forced to return to a body that fails me daily. I have struggled with random recurrent bowel obstructions since my J-pouch surgery. They can occur with something as simple as drinking water too fast or eating something my body can't digest, like raw carrots. I never know when it will happen. I can go months without one only to have two within a few weeks. The pain and nausea are crippling, and I spend hours in a fetal position as the pain passes through me in waves. I only move when I need to vomit. Once the obstruction clears, I can only drink fluids and eat simple foods, like toast and buttered noodles, for the next three to four days. Honestly, I would rather give birth to twins without an epidural than deal with an obstruction. I will vomit so often that I pass out from dehydration. I have been told that once this happens, I will need to go to a hospital for IV fluids and possible surgery, especially if the obstruction lasts more than twenty-four hours. My longest obstruction lasted seventeen and was beyond miserable. For this reason, I am careful what I eat, and, as mentioned, I have not had movie theater popcorn in twenty-five years—one of the saddest injustices of my life. In spite of these setbacks, I live a mostly normal life. Then again, how normal is life without popcorn?

I spend large amounts of time in nature, where I feel the closest connection to heaven possible while on Earth. As my now-strong legs carry me up winding mountain trails, the chaos of the city fades and I leave the noise behind, replaced by the crunch of dry leaves under my hiking boots. As I ascend, the air grows cooler, scented with pine sap and wildflowers. The sunlight filters through the canopy of trees and dances on the forest floor.

I shed the weight of the world, each step leaving me feeling lighter.

The rush of the river as it flows by, almost in a delicate dance, feels gloriously alive, healing me once again, and I feel some of the peace and love that engulfed me when I was out of my body.

I pause for a moment and close my eyes. The sun warms my soul, and a gentle breeze brushes my cheek. For a breathless moment, I am between two worlds again. It's not just a memory. It is a presence. It is love, longing, and joy, but most of all acceptance. An all-encompassing knowing that God has put me exactly where I am meant to be.

It is as if the universe is saying, "You are not alone."

I fight back the tears. I feel the connection, the veil between the seen and the unseen so thin.

It's easy to overlook the daily gifts of life. We live in such a hurried culture.

I encourage you to pause each day. Smell the fresh rain from a recent thunderstorm. Let the heat of a sunrise warm your soul. Stop and smell the flowers blooming in spring. These are all gentle reminders that heaven is near.

Sometimes all it takes is a minute of stillness to strengthen your connection with the divine.

Chapter 40

Eye See You, Trauma

In January 2023, I decided to do eye movement desensitization and reprocessing therapy (EMDR) to help me heal from some of the scarier memories of my time in the ICU, especially those of my abusive nurse. I had nightmares about Horrible Harlan, and some of those included reliving the painful procedures and surgeries I endured. I experienced the burning pain in my stomach and many of the moments under anesthesia, which I later verified through the medical records I requested in 2023. I woke up screaming, shaking, and dripping sweat, and the memories kept me up for hours because the pain felt so real. I wanted to take back some control of my feelings and rid myself of the nightmares.

I completed a year of weekly therapy with a wonderful therapist who patiently encouraged me to fully feel my feelings. It was not easy. It brought back memories I thought I could escape the same way I once thought I could go to a family Christmas party. On the days I sat in the chair with tears rolling down my cheeks, I wondered if I could truly heal.

It was a long and tiring process, but I am proud to say that when I think of the moments that used to terrify me when this monster of a nurse was present, I now see a small and feeble person who no longer holds power over me. He no longer lives in the shadows of my memories or takes up space that does not belong to him.

I can now walk into a hospital without losing my mind when I hear the beeping sounds of the equipment. I no longer feel the urge to throw up or pass out when I smell the strong scent of the alcohol swab pads used to sanitize my central and PICC lines. I don't panic when I get sick and need to see a doctor for a high fever or a simple sickness, fearing I will be admitted and spend months in critical care.

Instead, I think of the quieter, softer memories of my hospitalization—watching movies on the TV and VCR, or seeing the newborn babies through the nursery window as my family wheeled my wheelchair to the fourth floor.

Over time, the hospital transformed into something more than just a place of pain and survival. It became sacred.

Within those sterile walls, I crossed the veil between this life and the Other Side. I felt the presence of God and angels. I experienced healing not just of the body, but of the spirit. What was once a place of trauma became holy ground—a space where heaven touched earth, and where my soul was forever changed.

This journey of healing has helped me appreciate the impact our thoughts and actions have on our friends, family, and even strangers. We never know what another person is going through on any given day. They may have lost a loved one, been diagnosed with a debilitating disease, lost their job, fought with their spouse, or they may be caring for a parent in bad health. They may be lonely and not want to be on this earth anymore. We just don't know because many people put on a happy face in public. It could be that your offer to hold the door for someone struggling with their groceries may be the one good part of their day.

Live each day with intention and love. Smile at those you pass on the street. Let a car merge even if they waited until the last minute to get over and you feel like screaming at them and running them off the road. Bring flowers to a widowed neighbor and let them tell you about their sweetheart, whom they miss with all of their being. Help a single mom snow-blow her driveway in the winter or mow her lawn in the summer.

I truly feel if everyone found a way to bring more love and quit spreading hate and divisiveness, we could raise the collective love frequency many feel is missing. Love is not just a feeling—it's a force that heals, connects, and transforms us.

Chapter 41

Losing Diane: The Final Hug

On January 12, 2024, exactly twenty-four years after my soul left my body, I was allowed to feel heaven again.

It had been years since my illness, and now a very close friend, Diane, had slipped into a coma after complications during heart surgery.

Every waking moment of the two previous days, the grief of this new loss engulfed me. The heaviness was overpowering, and I cried continually.

I stared at my computer screen at work but couldn't focus. I picked up my phone to call or text Diane as usual, and then put it down when I remembered she could not answer.

When my mom and I visited her in the ICU, I knew her soul was not in her body. I could feel her off to the left beside her bed, next to the window. The loud, jarring noises of the machines keeping her alive transported me back to my time in the ICU, though not as triggering or traumatic. Her condition was critical. I put my hand over hers and told her how much her friendship meant to me. I knew that even though she was not awake, she felt my love. She was one of the first few people outside my family I had told about my divorce. Her warm hugs and unwavering support became an anchor, pulling me through some of my darkest moments. She had also separated from her husband when her kids were younger and knew the right words to say and even made me laugh. That shared vulnerability brought us closer. We developed an unshakable bond. She nicknamed my ex-husband "the puke." Over the years, she took my kids under her wing and loved them as her own. She made sure teenage Isaac always had spending money by hiring him to do her summer yard work. Sienna, who is a fierce carnivore, learned that Diane always had shrimp for her when cooking her Southern meals on Sundays. Her house smelled of heavenly jambalaya with rice that included an entire stick of butter. Diane and I took cooking classes at Williams Sonoma and grew veggies in our backyard gardens. In the winter, we bundled in coats, hopped in my car, and drove through neighborhoods admiring festive Christmas lights and décor, the streets transformed into a magical wonderland. Her eyes lit up each time we passed a house.

She had been raised in a military family and traveled all over the world, living in many foreign countries. Sienna loved to hear her talk about Japan since she had that trip on her bucket list.

Over fourteen years, we spent thousands of hours sitting on her front porch in rocking chairs, watching breathtaking pink-and-gold sunsets, talking about life, and laughing until our stomachs hurt. She was a dog person through and through befriending every neighborhood pup who strolled by with its human.

We giggled over stories of wild Mardi Gras parties and the men she dated during her college years at Louisiana State University. I'd fill her in on the misery of dating as a divorced woman in her thirties—if you've had that privilege, you understand. Diane and I would critique my dates and give them ridiculous nicknames, laughing until we cried.

Her imagination and storytelling made me feel like I was right there with her—in her LSU dorm room, or walking the steep hills of Japan, where she once lived with her husband and two small children. She welcomed me into her world without hesitation, openly sharing her dreams, memories, and even her deepest insecurities.

Sometimes she sat on her porch at night and shined a flashlight across the street into my bedroom window, which was directly across from her house.

"Heather," I'd hear her yell. "Come porch!"

"I'll be right there," I'd yell back as I ran across the street in my pajamas and bare feet, grinning like a child.

I'm sure we kept the neighbors up with our loud laughter. We'd stay out until the sky was so dark the only light came from the moon and the stars. She made me forget all my worries. It felt magical.

Her personality was larger than life.

Seeing her so lifeless was devastating.

On the night of the twelfth, I woke from a deep sleep. I lay on my side, facing the window, then rolled onto my back and stared at the ceiling, my house quiet. Suddenly, a warm feeling of love began to hover near the top of my head. It slowly traveled down my body, filling every inch of me until it reached my feet. It slowly surrounded my entire being, starting at one point and moving in a circle before connecting at another, like a round bubble, encompassing my body with light and vibrating energy. As this warmth passed through me, my grief disappeared, replaced by an enormous wave of healing. I felt my profound sadness change to acceptance. I floated in a sea of endless, energetic love. I looked at my clock to see it was 1:11 a.m. This time is significant to me because I see 11, 111, and 1,111 every single day in the most random places, and Diane knew this. It had been a joke between us how often the numbers appeared in my life.

As I basked in this feeling, I thanked God for allowing me to experience this profound act of compassion from Diane. It felt just like my time on the Other Side. This love was infinite, and I was able to stop crying and feel comfort and even joy. Like waves, that love and warmth washed over me again and again as I thought of my friend.

After an hour, I fell back asleep and dreamed of her. In this dream, I was at the hospital with my mom, visiting her. Diane sat next to me. Her soft smile reminded me of someone who had been told a fun secret and was eager to share it. She had a beautiful glow about her and appeared healthy and strong, unlike in life where she battled cancer and heart problems. She didn't need her oxygen to breathe, and she wasn't worn down by her health or the long hours at her job.

She telepathically communicated to me that she had gone to heaven and "had seen God and beautiful mountains and more."

I felt honored that she had shared this with me. I told her I wanted to hear everything once she was home from the hospital. I told her we needed to write down her experience so she could read it after she healed. Still in the dream, I went into the hallway to a café just past the nurses' desk outside her room. I asked the cashier/barista for a pen and paper and took them back to the room.

As I sat down next to Diane, my Spirit Guide told me Diane would be the one to make the decision to return to her body or not. I knew whatever she decided would be right for her. I was then told I would be okay either way. I would have the peace of knowing she would be close and watch over me if she stayed there.

This dream comforted me and gave me permission to move through each day focusing on happier memories instead of being stuck in the painful ones, which were paralyzing.

After my dream, when I went to visit Diane in the ICU, I could feel her excitement and anticipation about going back *home* again.

Instead of crying or fearing what might happen, I knew she would be with me even if in a different form. I didn't need to worry about what she decided because love is energy, and energy never dies.

Ultimately, Diane passed away on January 15, never having woken up from her coma. She suffered a horrible death as the life-support machines slowly shut down. Knowing that someone I loved was slipping away and I couldn't stop it was a moment I would like to forget. I miss her every day.

I know when my time comes to return to my loved ones, she will be there to greet me and welcome me back with a "Hi, hun" in her sweet Southern accent.

Whenever I am having a sad moment, I remember an insight Diane shared with me when I was going through a hard time. "How do you eat an elephant? One bite at a time." This helps me remember not to get overwhelmed when things feel too big and scary. I can take a deep breath and know that, at the end of the day, I *will* be okay.

Since her passing, I have felt Diane many, many times. She always announces her presence with love and joy. It brings me to tears to feel her so close to me once again. As promised, her influence from the other side has been monumental, and I continue to be on the receiving end of incredible gifts from her.

Two days before she went into surgery, I went to visit her at her house to help her get ready. She was a devout Catholic who sometimes had very strong promptings about her life. "I don't have a good feeling about this surgery. I had a dream that I'm going to die and my friend Katie, who will be at the hospital when it happens, will plan my funeral," she said.

"Diane! Don't you dare leave me!" I told her as I put my hand on her arm to give her a quick squeeze of love. I couldn't imagine life without her.

Diane looked scared. "What if it does happen?"

The room felt heavy with emotion. I wanted to tell her she couldn't go, couldn't leave me. "Well," I said, trying to keep my voice steady, "I will come take your beloved Margaritaville beach-cruiser bike and ride it around the neighborhood as I yell at the sky for you to come back." It was a long-running joke between us—the adorable mint-green bike with pineapple drink holder and wicker basket.

For months, she had been sick with cancer and heart issues. She had bought the bike the previous summer, but it sat in her garage, unused, the tags still on it. She had become weaker recently, requiring oxygen. When we sat on the porch, we daydreamed of the day she was healthy and we could ride bikes together.

"If you do die, you better fix my stomach and send me lots of money," I said, only half joking. She saw me at my worst and knew how much pain my hundreds of bowel obstructions caused. She promised to help me from the Other Side, making sure to visit me, maybe even yell boo! I told her I couldn't lose her and to please come home as soon as she could.

We spent the rest of the evening together. I helped her clean her kitchen while her beloved LSU football team played on the TV in the background. Every Sunday, I helped her with her house chores while we talked and gossiped. It was a familiar and comforting routine. As I left to go home for the night, I hugged and told her I loved her. She told me to be careful as I ran across the icy street to my house. I didn't realize that would be the last time I saw her. If I had known, I would have run back and given her one more big hug, wrapping her tightly in my arms, not letting go. I would have told her again how her friendship saved me. I know, though, that she knew my heart and felt my love and friendship.

A few weeks after her funeral, I woke up in the morning, and my stomach did not hurt. Until this point, I'd had a total of three pain-free days in twenty-five years. Anytime I ate, I had belly pain, so not having this pain was a shockingly different way to start my day. I went about my day thinking how cool it was that my entire day didn't revolve around the constant throbbing in my lower abdomen where my J-pouch was. And as the days went on, I stayed free of pain. It is actually real, the relief, not imaginary or temporary.

This gift from Diane is one I never thought was possible. I could never imagine life without pain. I continue to feel 95 percent better, and my outlook on life has never been so optimistic. I call her my magical friend and am grateful beyond words that she took my joke seriously and granted my wish.

In the summer months, you will find me riding Diane's beach cruiser around the neighborhood. Her daughter gifted it to me on the day of her funeral. As the wind flows through my hair, I imagine Diane clinging to the back of the bike as we fly down the street together. For those few moments, I forget that she is not waiting for me on her porch when I return home.

Chapter 42

Soul Contracts and Other Pre-Earth Goodies

My journey post-NDE has brought people into my life that I know without a doubt were meant to play a part in my story.

I don't believe in fate so much as I think we all have a plan and are given certain gifts and experiences to help guide us until we graduate and return home. I now have a more profound appreciation of life and feel an urgency to fully experience every moment life offers. I have found that to reach my goals, I sleep less and push my body more. I have a renewed sense of purpose and know there are tasks I must still complete. I love stronger and feel others' emotions on a higher level, which is both a curse and a blessing. Human connection is crucially important because everyone wants to feel included and acknowledged.

Although I am thankful for my second chance, I would be lying if I didn't admit that I crave being on the Other Side and feeling that vibrant, absolute love. I cannot put into words how hard it has been to be fully in this world every day. The magnetic pull of the Other Side and my daily struggle to feel fully present in this earthly realm are real.

Sometimes I think about how ridiculous this life is. Each day, we go to work and do the same boring tasks. I find myself thinking how silly it is that we place emphasis on things that do not really matter in this life. We fight wars with hate when love and communication could solve so many arguments. We spend so much of our waking hours not really experiencing life.

The divorce rate for couples where one partner experiences an NDE is 65 percent. I became that statistic. Even though I really loved Matt, I knew our goals were different, and deep in my soul, something felt off. Because he didn't experience the profoundly beautiful moments I did, he couldn't fully understand them when I shared what I experienced. For him and my family, especially my mom, my hospitalization was incredibly traumatic, and there were no "feel-good" moments. When I talked about my extraordinary experiences, he listened, but I think that, eventually, it was easier for him to move on and leave that part of his life behind.

Someone who glimpses the Other Side comes back changed in a way that's hard to articulate because there are no words for what they've experienced. Our earthly vocabulary can't begin to describe what we have felt. I think of it like a large radio tower with different frequencies; if you are tuned to a different radio station than someone else, they can't hear what you are listening to.

Nothing on this earth compares to my glimpse of the Other Side. Nothing. I have spoken to many individuals who had NDEs who don't feel like they fit into society anymore. Many times, I will notice that while I am in a crowded room, I feel like I am watching from the sidelines, not fully present. It is confusing. I sometimes feel isolated because I belong to two worlds and neither can fully hold me.

In 2023, I joined the board of directors for the Utah Chapter of IANDS, the International Association for Near-Death Studies. Each month, we have a speaker who's had an NDE. Although many of their experiences differ vastly from mine, we share that same knowledge of the overwhelming love and compassion that exists on the Other Side. They, too, know there is not another earthly experience that matches what they have seen and felt—not the birth of their first baby, not their favorite vacation, not a stunning sunrise, not even the pure joy of a child's laughter. Nothing.

This doesn't mean life is devoid of emotion and love for someone who's experienced an NDE; it just means we've seen colors that don't exist in this realm, basked in the freedom of being outside our bodies, witnessed indescribable moments of beauty, and now have the divine *knowledge* that life continues beyond what we see.

Our soul is a fire that can never be extinguished.

Life on the Other Side is more vivid and alive than life on this earth. If I could pass on only one thing I learned from my time there, it is that we need to love more fiercely and create a life we can look back on and be proud of.

In August 2024, I attended the annual international five-day IANDS conference in Phoenix, Arizona, with around seven hundred other people. I was surrounded by individuals who had also experienced near-death or spiritually transformative experiences (STE) or were interested in learning more about otherworldly things.

This was a life-changing, love-filled experience, and I wanted to bask in it forever. For the first time in almost twenty-five years, I sat with those who didn't need to communicate with words because our souls connected on a higher plane of energy. My entire being felt energized and in tune with the Other Side on a level that had been missing as I went through the motions of daily life.

I wanted to stay here forever, cocooned in the bliss of being understood, surrounded by a symphony of souls vibrating at the same harmonious frequency. I wanted to spread this energy to the world and let everyone else experience what happens when you let down your walls and gather together as souls who come from the same loving home.

I came home with a renewed sense of purpose that set me on a course I never would have imagined for myself.

I am looking forward to where this journey takes me as my guide continues to whisper to my soul each time I need him.

I have been given a second chance. I should not have survived my illness and death, and I understand the magnitude of that gift on a profound level. I am overwhelmingly thankful I was entrusted with these experiences and for the difference they've made in my life.

Chapter 43

Dr. Jeff

When I arrived at the hospital on December, 20, 1999, Dr. Jeff O'Driscoll was my attending ER physician. With input from another doctor, he decided to admit me. I know without a doubt that his decision saved my life.

If I had been sent home that day with orders to follow up with my gastroenterologist, I would not be alive today. My denial was so intense that even as I faced death, I really thought I was going to be okay if I could just get my fevers under control. I am sure I downplayed my symptoms as he checked me over. He could have easily agreed with me, but based on my symptoms and the paperwork from previous ER visits, he chose a different path. After he admitted me, we went our separate ways, and I doubt he ever thought of me again. I forgot his name as I began my journey to death and back.

In 2023, I unknowingly had dinner with a group of NDE experiencers and sharers. Dr. O'Driscoll was part of that group.

I again ran into him a year later at the IANDS conference in Phoenix. My guide literally pushed me forward to go talk to him when I saw him standing alone during an end-of-conference party (which I almost didn't attend). As we talked, he told me he had been a doctor at the same hospital I was at. We made plans to meet for lunch when we were both back in town so he could hear about my experiences. I still did not realize he was a significant part of my past.

He listened intently as I talked about my story. He asked what had made me talk to him at the conference, and I told him how I felt pushed forward by my guide.

We stayed in touch, and one night as I read through my medical records, I saw his name as the attending physician involved in my care. I felt the air leave my lungs as I stared at the paperwork. I do not believe in coincidences. My guide brought us together again, twenty-five years later, for a reason.

Since my NDE, many doctors and nurses have come to realize that it's actually very common for a critical patient to leave their body and travel to the Other Side. Many have started asking their patients if they've had any unusual experiences they would like to talk about. I believe that as society becomes more understanding and begins to allow survivors to tell their stories, those too scared to speak will come forward. Profoundly beautiful stories are waiting to be told. I look forward to meeting new friends who have had similar moments that reshaped their lives, bringing them the knowledge that each and every one of us on this earth matters and that we are here to bring light and love to all.

Chapter 44

Love Is the Greatest Gift

What I have learned from my time on the Other Side is that the most important gift is to show love and compassion to others. Love is the fundamental reason for everything, a force that drives us and connects us. It's a simple but profound truth: treat others the way you want to be treated. In this life, everyone is fighting some type of battle, even if behind closed doors. All too often, I see people hide behind religion as their "return ticket" to heaven. During my time on the Other Side, I found no divisions, no boundaries between people based on religion, race, or gender. Rather, the universal language of unconditional love transcended the divisions we place on ourselves. What matters is the love we carry in our hearts and how we treat one another.

Sometimes we are conditioned as children to have prejudices about others, those prejudices getting in the way of loving those we deem inferior. Or we have enemies we cannot possibly love. In these moments, we can pray for them if we are unable to do anything else.

We all originate from the same source, each of us with a unique purpose. That purpose begins with love. It encompasses many sacred talents we were sent here with to help guide us home. Whether that talent is service, compassion, music, intelligence, or even just being a good friend who shows up when someone feels alone, every act of love sends a ripple of positive, healing energy. And the more of that energy we put out into the universe, the more love will be returned to us. Each day in our lives counts; even the most mundane day is important in our quest to return to the Other Side. I am humbled by these precious moments I experienced and feel so honored that I can share them with those open to and seeking this love and knowledge.

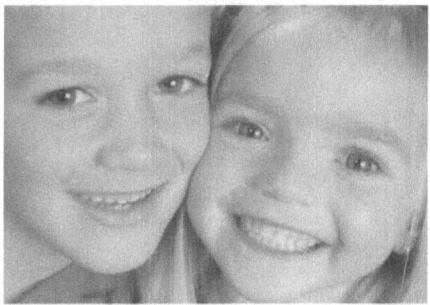

My precious little ones.

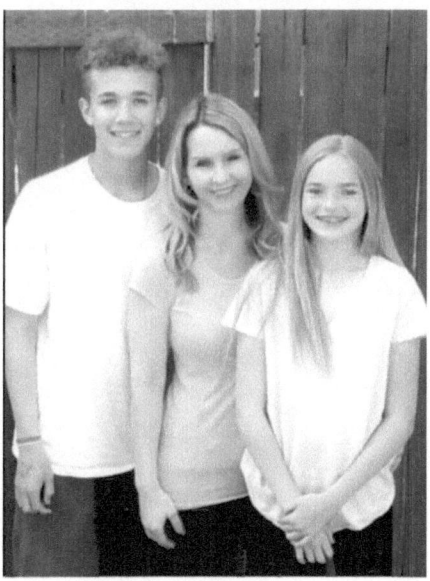

My children, my greatest gifts.

A Mystery Unveiled

W hen this book was first published, I did not yet know the identity of the man in the top hat.

The story you are about to read unfolded after publication. It felt important to include it here, as it answers a question I carried for twenty-five years.

Some answers arrive in their own time.

Chapter 45

Through Generations

For twenty-five years, I wondered about the man in the top hat. Who was he? Although he felt unknown, he was also deeply familiar. The moment I saw him, I felt safe. His dark, soulful eyes burned into my memory. Over the years, I thought of him at unexpected times, unsettled that I had no answer for who he was. Maybe he was one of my guides. Maybe he was the one assigned to usher souls through the tunnel at their passing.

Then one day in 2025, I received the answer I had been waiting for.

My second cousin Linda, the daughter of my grandmother's sister, had listened to an interview I did with a well-known podcaster. In it, I described the man in the top hat. Shortly after, she sent me a message.

"I'm so excited to see that you are finally getting your story out there. Congrats! My mom once told me about a dream she had years ago. A man in a top hat told her she looked just like her mother. She always felt it was her grandpa George, who had mysteriously disappeared. Did you ever find out who the man was?"

I read the message once. Then I read it again.

A man in a top hat?

My great-great grandfather George?

A mysterious disappearance?

Could it possibly be the same person?

It seemed impossible. I had never seen a photograph of him. I knew very little about him. But I love a good mystery, and I was intrigued. I called my mom and told her we were about to go on a family history adventure. My goal was simple. Find a photograph. Put twenty-five years of questions to rest.

As we searched through online genealogy records, his name appeared on the screen. I held my breath as I read. In our family, his story ended abruptly. He left one day for work and never returned. No one ever knew what happened.

Below his story were two grainy photographs from the 1800s.

Time stopped.

I was looking into the eyes of the man who had stood with me as my soul left my body. The man who had waited in the tunnel, steady and protective, ready to guide me home.

I did not have words.

I never expected to see my protector again, yet here he was, staring back at me while I sat in my parents' living room. I zoomed in on the image on my phone. He was not wearing a top hat in the photograph, and he did not have a beard. But the eyes. The bone structure. The expression.

It was him. I would recognize his face anywhere.

For twenty-five years, I wondered who stood between me and the light at the end of the tunnel.

It was a man who had vanished one day, leaving my great-grandmother without a father. A man whose story never had an ending. A mystery that was never solved.

And somehow, across generations, across time, across whatever separates this world from the next, he was there when I needed comfort most.

I do not know why he appeared to me in that dark tunnel. I do not know whether he was there to guide me home or simply to remind me that I come from people who endure the unexplainable.

Maybe what awaits us on the Other Side is not just a destination.

Maybe it is a thread woven through generations, through memory, through moments we only understand years later.

I am reminded again of the Chinese proverb:

"An invisible red thread connects those who are destined to meet, regardless of time, place, or circumstance. The thread may stretch or tangle, but it will never break."

I came back to finish my story, a story intertwined with those who came before me and those who will come after.

The man in the top hat is no longer a mystery.

He is family.

I was never alone.

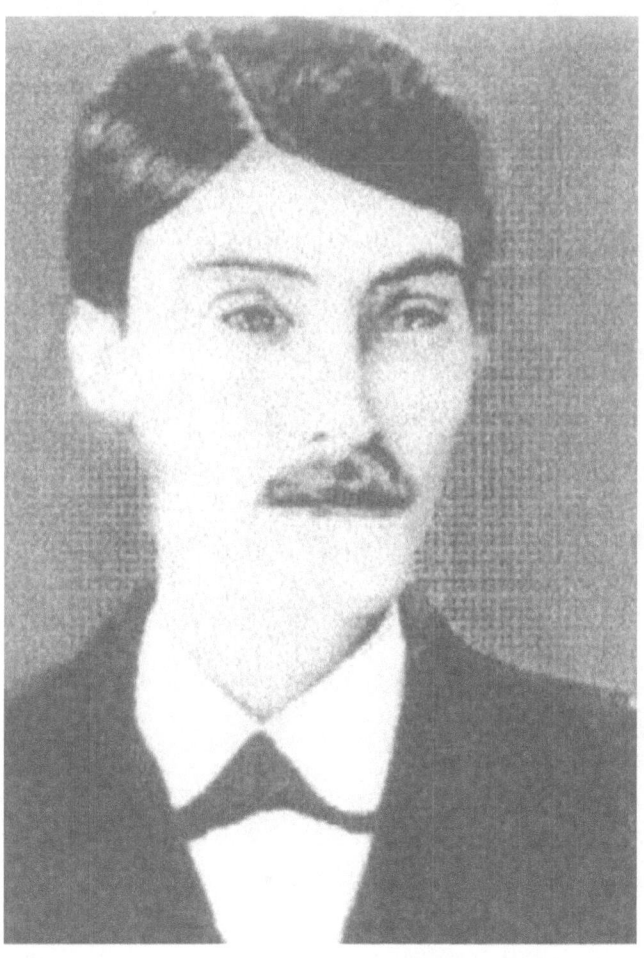

Acknowledgments

It has been said that raising a child takes a village. Writing this book was no different, and I am deeply thankful for my village. While there are too many people who have been a part of my life journey to include here, I would be ungrateful if I didn't thank a select few who contributed profoundly to shaping my life in such a positive way.

To my parents, Craig and Rosemary: There are no words that can truly capture how much your love and support have meant to me. You never gave up on me, no matter how difficult the road became. You walked with me through every twist and turn, facing life's challenges with me side by side. Your unwavering belief in me, especially when I doubted myself, has been a guiding light in my journey. The sacrifices you made while I was in the hospital, dropping everything to care for me, fight for me, and hold me through my darkest days—those acts of love saved my life. Even now you continue to love and protect me, and I will carry that love with me forever, always.

To my brothers, Josh and Shawn: Your constant love and protection throughout the years have been a blessing beyond measure. You've always been there for me in ways both big and small, and I'm incredibly lucky to have you both in my life. Thank you for giving me the joy of being surrounded by the best nephews and niece anyone could ask for. Being Aunt Heather is a gift I hold dear. I am forever grateful for the unwavering bond we share.

To Tori: I cherished every single minute of being your mama. You were my heart's greatest joy, and the love I have for you is immeasurable. My sweet baby girl, you will always have a sacred place in my heart, a space that is yours and yours alone. No matter where life leads me, I will carry your love with me forever.

To Isaac and Sienna, my beautiful children: Thank you for the extraordinary gift of allowing me to be your mother. Through sleepless nights, laugh-out-loud moments, whispered prayers, and the quiet, ordinary moments in between—you have filled my life with purpose and joy. I hope that as you look back on the memories we've created, you'll feel the depth of my love in every one of them. To the moon and back and then even further—always.

To Breezi Ainsworth: Thank you for your unwavering love and support and for the countless hours you spent by my side in the hospital. Our many years of friendship have been a gift I cherish more than words can express. Even when we're apart, always know that you are deeply loved and forever in my heart.

To Diane Burandt: There are no words to fully capture how deeply I miss you. Your absence is felt every day, and yet I take comfort in knowing you are watching over me and my children from above. Your love continues to guide me even from the Other Side. Until the day I see you again, save me a seat on your porch, my dear friend. I carry you in my heart always.

To Brian Anthony: Your friendship means more to me than words can say. Thank you for your constant encouragement and for filling my life with laughter through this wild journey we call life. I truly couldn't have done this without you by my side.

To Jenny Johnson, Lee Smith, and Valerie Sorensen: Your support during my divorce was nothing short of monumental. Those Friday night dinners filled with laughter that lifted the heaviness from my heart were more than a tradition—they were therapy. In your presence, my broken soul found comfort and healing. Thank you, my dear friends, for carrying me through.

To Martin Tanner: Thank you for your unwavering support as I shared my story. I am deeply grateful not only for your wisdom but for the genuine friendship we share. Our conversations are a gift I always look forward to, filled with insight and connection. Your encouragement has meant more to me than words can fully express. You've had a monumental influence on my journey—beginning with the moment you first encouraged me to share my story openly—and your friendship has been a constant source of strength along the way.

To Lynn Taylor: It was very healing to put the pen to paper and write what has been patiently waiting for over twenty-five years to be shared. Thank you for nudging me to write this book. It is scary to put myself out there with something so personal, but your encouragement and help every step of the way was priceless in creating this memoir.

To Richard Paul Evans: Thank you for being both a mentor and an inspiration. Your generous support and the wisdom you so willingly shared gave me the foundation I needed to bring this book to life. Your guidance and advice were monumental as I poured my heart into a book that might never have been written. In moments of doubt, your belief in my voice helped steady my resolve. Because of you, I found the strength and courage to tell my story with vulnerability, honesty, and hope.

To my editor, Zina Petersen: Thank you from the bottom of my heart. You didn't just polish my words; you helped me find my voice. In a story born of pain, your guidance made space for moments of light, grace, and even laughter. You saw through the sorrow and reminded me that my spirit and my story could still shine. This book would not be what it is without your intuition, encouragement, and unwavering belief in my voice. I am forever grateful.

To my editor, Michele Priesendorf: I believe without a doubt that we were brought together for a reason. In the midst of your own journey through grief, you gave this story such care and presence. Thank you for walking this path with me—your strength and compassion have left a lasting imprint on both this book and my heart.

To Aunt Lucille: Thank you for believing in this book before it ever existed. Every time we saw each other, you would gently ask, "Have you started writing yet?"—and your quiet persistence stayed with me long after. You planted the seed, and I carried your encouragement through every word. These pages are my quiet answer to your loving question.

To Jo Agnew: Whether it's hiking adventures or fun times with Diane, some of my favorite memories are with you. Aren't you glad you took a chance on me, despite my legendary RBF? Love you massive, my dear friend.

To Jaimie Graham: From pink sparkles to flowers, and all things pretty, you just… get me. Thank you for adding so much sweetness—literally and figuratively—to my life. You're a great partner in crime… er, I mean, in design.

About the Author

Heather Vandermeyden never imagined her twenties would be spent in a fight for her life. After a sudden and severe medical crisis left her in the ICU for months, she lost the ability to walk, talk, and care for herself. But what began as a battle for survival became the beginning of a deeper spiritual awakening. During this time, Heather experienced a series of profound near-death experiences that revealed glimpses of the afterlife, the presence of divine love, and a healing purpose greater than she had ever known.

The journey back was long—physically, emotionally, and spiritually—but it was also sacred. With each step, Heather began to rebuild not only her body but her entire life, guided by the wisdom she brought back from beyond.

Today, Heather shares her extraordinary story to audiences across the country, offering hope to those who are grieving, healing, or searching for meaning. She serves as a board member of the Utah Chapter of the International Association for Near-Death Studies (IANDS), where she helps build a community of spiritual seekers and experiencers. Her voice carries the quiet authority of someone who has touched the eternal—and returned with a message.

Heather is also a mother to two children she first met during her time beyond this world. She finds daily joy in hiking the nearby mountains, paddle boarding, interior design and the simple, sacred beauty of life after death—and life after survival.

Learn more at heathervandermeyden.com.

www.ingramcontent.com/pod-product-compliance
Lightning Source LLC
Chambersburg PA
CBHW031509120626
46545CB00005B/1800